Sex is
a
Four-Letter Word

Dr Sudhakar Krishnamurti is an internationally renowned andrologist and microsurgeon, and the first Indian doctor to practise exclusive clinical andrology — the branch of medicine that deals with disorders of the male reproductive system. Dr Krishnamurti is the only Asian to have ever won the prestigious Herbert Newman international award for original clinical research in the field of sexual medicine. He won this for having described the 'Krishnamurti Operation' for a condition called Peyronie's disease. Dr Krishnamurti is also the only Indian in his field to have been twice appointed on W.H.O. international experts' committees. He is presently the director of Andromeda Andrology Centre, Hyderabad, India, the country's first andrology centre.

Dr Krishnamurti is also a popular columnist and writer who is known for his tongue-in-cheek brand of medical humour. Over the years, he has written for many newspapers, periodicals, ezines and web portals by invitation. *The Times of India, The Asian Age, India Today Plus, The Week, Femina, Deccan Chronicle, Business in Thailand* are a few. He also contributes regularly to medical textbooks and journals, and lectures and demonstrates surgery all over the world.

Dr Krishnamurti lives in Hyderabad with his paediatrician wife Kiran, and their two daughters, Ulrika and Aria. *Sex Is Not A Four Letter Word* is his first book.

Contents

Foreword

In the 1970s film, *Sleeper*, there is a scene where Woody Allen is in the operation theatre, awaiting brain surgery following a head injury. Just before he is administered anaesthesia, he requests the neurosurgeon to take especial care of his brain. 'The brain's my second favourite organ, doc,' he says, matter-of-factly. No prizes, of course, for guessing what Allen's favourite organ is. Woody's favourite is my favourite too. The only difference is that his is avocational whereas mine's vocational.

Hence this book.

This work has no literary pretensions whatsoever. It is a plain-speaking and sincere attempt to draw the readers' attention to my chosen field of andrology and sexual medicine. It is written as much for the reader with a healthy curiosity about sexual matters as for the millions out there — male, female, intersex and transsexual — who suffer from some sexual problem or the other, and for those who live with or know someone who does.

The term *andrology* is unknown to most. For some obscure reason, the Greek root 'gynaik', which means 'woman', seems to be familiar to many. Yet 'andrology', with its exactly identical and obvious Greek roots, is something that even most doctors haven't heard of. What's worse is that many dictionaries don't mention it either. This is despite Google and Yahoo yielding nearly 800,000 links (at the time of writing) when one enters 'andrology' as the search term. *Blakiston's Medical Dictionary* defines andrology as, 'The science of diseases of the male sex, especially of those of the male reproductive organs.' Etymologically, 'andro' is a combining form which means 'male', 'male part or organ'. Yet, though its analogue — gynaecology — has been established as a discipline for centuries now, the birth of andrology is relatively recent.

I have been practising clinical andrology for the past twenty years.

The most important reason for andrology's relative obscurity was the erroneous belief, both within and outside the scientific community, that all sexual problems in human males lay 'between the ears'. Scientists knew long ago that complex neuromuscular, vascular and other phenomena are involved in the physical act of raising of a human finger, for instance, yet they illogically supposed that the raising of a human penis was totally psychologically mediated and, that all it took to raise it was a naughty thought. Thus, for a long time, all sexual problems remained in the realm of psychology and psychiatry. It took medical science a few centuries to prove this belief wrong. Today, at last, it is finally well known that in nearly eighty to ninety per cent of cases of persistent impotence (erectile dysfunction, ED) in men, the cause is physical, or organic, rather than psychological, or functional.

The other important reason for the delay is male chauvinism. Historically, men have been notorious for their refusal to admit to sexual inadequacies. In the old, male-dominated patriarchal societies, it was quite common for a man to label a woman 'barren' if he couldn't sire a child, or call her 'frigid' when it was, in fact, he who was impotent. Men sometimes divorced several wives using this unfair, unscientific and arbitrary 'diagnosis'. The prospect of a man going to a physician to have his manhood checked out was unthinkable. The few that did go ended up being told that it was 'all in the mind', or fell victims to quacks and charlatans and their futile ministrations.

The emergence of the Gloria Steinems and the Lorena Bobbitts has changed all this forever. Today, few women will suffer a partner's impotence or low sperm counts silently. The New Age woman will dare her man to prove that he is man enough, or will force him to seek treatment, leave him or even seek greener pastures. Women are increasingly addressing their sexual needs and problems emphatically nowadays. FSD, or Female Sexual Dysfunction, has become a big thing. Not so long ago, all this was quite unthinkable.

Incidentally, have you ever noticed that women are much less reluctant and inhibited than men when it comes to seeking medical attention for reproductive system-related complaints? A woman will go to her gynaecologist with her husband, her boyfriend, her father, her brother even. She sees nothing wrong in it. She is not embarrassed. She does not hide her face or peer over her shoulder. Even women seeking termination of unwanted pregnancies out of wedlock come straight to the point nowadays. In my office, I have women openly talking about their orgasms, and about what sexual stimulation they'd like to receive during love-making.

The wheel has come full circle. Men better understand this in a hurry, or else.

Some years ago, in 1994 to be precise, the World Health Organisation (WHO) declared sex a fundamental human health right and an important quality of life (QOL) health issue. This brought andrology and sexual medicine under the spotlight and kindled the attention of not only the medical fraternity, but also others, most notably industry and the media.

This has had both good and bad consequences. Concomitant with the tremendous advances in medical, pharmaceutical and bio-medical sexual research, there has also been a media explosion in the depiction of brazen sexuality and pornography. However, by no means is all the stuff out there on sex real and accurate. Much of it, in fact, can be damaging, especially to the young and impressionable, in whom the enthusiasm for sex is directly proportional to the colossal ignorance of the subject. Since they've never received any formal sex education, these youngsters (most adults, too) start to believe that pornography is synonymous with sex. This is very dangerous, as you will see in some of the stories inside this book.

Contemporary societal changes in sexual mores and practices also make a compelling case for dissemination of correct sex education. For instance, today we see more promiscuous single people, higher divorce–remarriage rates, a boom in adolescent sexual precocity, more extra-marital sex, homosexuals, lesbians and transsexuals coming out of the closet in droves, increased geriatric sexuality secondary to longevity and improved general health, the ogre of HIV/ AIDS, et cetera, than ever before. Nearly everybody receives tons of sexual spam in their email: one email message promises the most perverse and best multi-orgasmic cyber sex while another assures bucketfuls of ejaculate and longer, thicker penises. Our children are watching more of both, blatant as well as suggestive sex on TV than ever before. On the other hand, by stark contrast, our children note that their own parents at home seem, for the most part, to be quite asexual beings, and wonder why this is so. The child is confused. To make matters worse, the child receives no sex education to speak of, which could help put matters in perspective. Even the few antiseptic diagrams of the male and female genitalia shown in biology class in secondary school are thought to be too graphically sexual by our moralists and educationists. It's hardly surprising then that most kids obtain all their education from all the wrong sources. On the whole, the sexual 'literacy rates' in our society are pathetic, contrary to what you might imagine.

There are many 'sex education' books already out there. Unfortunately, many of these are like medical textbooks written for students to cram before an exam. Others have attempted to write guide-style ready reference manuals for lay people. These too have proved insipid and equally 'sexless'. Historically, books in these educational categories have been used more as trouble-shooters for those who face sexual problems of some sort, rather than pre-emptively as educational tools, to be read before one's initiation into sex. Thus, educational information about sex has always been treated as something dull that is meant only for the sexually inept or crippled, not as something that we all need in order to be able to lead healthy, normal and responsible sexual lives.

It is not surprising therefore, that the unreal, titillating sexual hype provided by pornography is so popular. We have already seen what damage that can do.

Thus, both the *establishment* (school curricula and other sex education tools) and the *anti-establishment* (pornography) sex education models have failed. Conventional sex education is inadequate and boring. Nobody wants it. By contrast, pornography is exciting, but miseducates and causes harm.

Hence, I felt that there is a definite place for a clean, *edutaining* sex education package, one that is both accurately educative and entertaining. If only sex were packaged right, I thought, we could contribute so much to societal and medical welfare with it. And this is what *Sex is Not a Four-Letter Word* attempts to do. However, I must hasten to add that this book has no intention whatsoever to be a comprehensive resource or reference book on the subject.

The following pages contain some short stories and essays, a few of which have appeared in some form in some columns and articles earlier written by me for newspapers, periodicals and e-zines. Many of these are true stories of patients whom I have actually encountered and treated successfully in the course of my private practice as a clinical andrologist over the past two decades. Failures have been omitted not because they don't occur in clinical practice but because the idea is to convey to readers what scientific knowledge has made possible. By the same token, if reference has been made to acts of omission or commission by colleagues, it is only from the standpoint of presenting the scientific facts and current position on a subject. There is no intention to disparage any specialist or specialty. Some of the contents of a few essays have been derived from some internet and other resources. These are presumed to be in the public information domain and there is no intention here to infringe on any copyright. Any inadvertent exception may kindly be brought to our attention.

Though the medical facts are authentic, some of the other details in the stories have been modified to make for better reading. I have taken the liberty of fictionalising and exaggerating some portions for effect. Some chapters are extrapolated from observations outside the medical setting. However, each essay draws attention to some andrological or other sexual matter, directly or indirectly, or narrates a case history. An attempt is made to infuse medical information into the fabric of the tale — in the same way that necessary, but bitter, medicine is often cloaked with sugar.

In order to retain the original context and a true-to-life feel, the stories have been sometimes told in the actual language used by the protagonists. Thus, the dialogue is sometimes colloquial, and the vocabulary sometimes colourful. No attempt has been made to change these. This is intentional and I am confident that even the purists among you will read it in the right spirit and not find anything really objectionable. Personally, I believe that the contents of this book are clean enough to even warrant its introduction as a recommended reading text for high school and college students. That is how much sex education information it contains between the lines. Who knows, with our present-day liberalised and modern leadership, this might happen sooner than we imagine. After all, the language employed here is no different than what the average student uses or encounters everyday in countless other books and media.

I sincerely hope that all of you will enjoy reading these stories and essays as much as I did writing them, and that, no matter how well informed you already are, you will still learn a new thing or two.

Dr Sudhakar Krishnamurti
[www.sudhakarkrishnamurti.com]

1

Mr Maggi Noodle

Some years ago, a battle-ax of a woman stormed into my office, wanting to discuss her husband's andrological problem. She didn't wait to be announced in by my secretary, or even knock on my door. She just blew the door open, stomped in, pulled up a chair on the other side of my desk, and plopped her bulk on to it. I could hear the poor chair creaking in protest. I pulled out my hanky and discreetly mopped the sudden sweat droplets that had appeared on my forehead. Such things don't happen to me every day.

Apparently, this shrew didn't believe in any foreplay or preliminaries. She nosedived straight to the point. 'You must help my husband, doc,' she thundered. 'He has a Maggi noodle problem.'

I wanted to guffaw out loud but forced myself to adopt a funereal demeanour instead, because this bazooka seemed dead serious. There are various flavours of Maggi noodles, I reminded her. Most of them are tasty. Also, a noodle is crisp to begin with, so where's the problem, I wanted to know. She seemed impressed by my earnestness and also by my vast knowledge of noodles, and proceeded to explain her husband's situation a little more elaborately.

'You are right about the "being crisp to begin with" part doc,' she conceded. 'But that's the problem. It remains crisp only for two minutes. I'm not even ready yet and it becomes limp. That's why I have named my husband the "Mr Two Minute Maggi Noodle Man". Everything's over in just two minutes.'

The thought did cross my mind that to last two entire minutes by the clock with this termagant, the guy must actually be quite a super stud or something, but I quickly quashed the unfair and unscientific thought and came back to the serious andrological matter at hand. I made a mental note to recommend Mr Maggi for a bravery award some day; if anybody ever asked me for nominations, that is.

'This Maggi noodle problem that you describe is very common, ma'am,' I told her, realising that I probably sounded more like an oriental chef than like an andrologist. 'But I can't help you unless I see your husband and get to the bottom of this,' I concluded, cleverly.

Thereupon, Mrs Maggi got up, walked to the door, leaned out, and crooked her index finger at somebody or something I couldn't see. The suspense was building up now and I couldn't wait to see this man — who sounded like he belonged more in a bowl of Chinese soup than in a bedroom. Soon, Mr Maggi walked in with a mixture of sheepishness and relief. The latter, I suspected, was because he was finally meeting a potential saviour who would help him avenge this harridan. I put out my chest, and slid my chair forward. I wanted my heart to reach out to him, and was determined to make him rise to the occasion.

The next several minutes were dead serious. I told Mr and Mrs Maggi to take it easy, that this is a very common problem, and an eminently curable one at that. I pointed out that above the age of forty, fifty per cent of men have some form of erectile dysfunction (ED) or impotence. This can manifest either as a reduction in rigidity, or as a sustenance problem, that is, the erections are fairly rigid to begin with, but the man is unable to maintain that rigidity. Sometimes, there is difficulty even in obtaining an erection. There are many risk factors and causes for this. Ageing, diabetes, high blood pressure (hypertension), high cholesterol levels, obesity, a sedentary lifestyle, hormonal changes accompanying ageing (andropause/male menopause), smoking, excessive drinking, to name a few common ones, can all cause erectile dysfunction.

In the case of the Maggis, it turned out that Mr Maggi did attain some kind of erection, though this was not as good as what he was capable of a few months ago. However, he couldn't sustain it, and would lose it soon after commencing intercourse. He was not a premature ejaculator though, and his wife's ranting and raving didn't seem to have much of a deleterious effect on his libido either. I once again thought of the bravery awards.

Investigation revealed that Mr Maggi had not just one, but all of the conditions listed above. He was 47, was detected to be both diabetic and hypertensive (with high blood pressure; hypertension does not mean a 'hyper' person or someone with too much 'tension') four years ago, and was on medication for these conditions. His was also a sedentary, high pressure job and he smoked incessantly. Further, he was obese and had never exercised in his life. To make matters worse, he partied four to five nights a week. I would have been surprised if this man *hadn't* had erectile dysfunction. His, in fact, is a classical case. What was unfortunate was that his physician never once warned him about the possibility of developing erectile dysfunction, even though he was treating Maggi for so many diseases that could cause it. It was even worse that Maggi never once mentioned his problem to his doctor either. It took a woman to finally address the matter.

Further tests focused closer on the erectile dysfunction. It turned out that Mr Maggi had only a sixty-seven per cent erection, which too he was not able to sustain for long. I put him on medication. These worked reasonably well for about two years, but he eventually opted for an operation because he did not want to take these drugs for indefinitely long periods. 'They are bound to have long-term side effects, doc,' he told me. 'Besides, they take away all spontaneity from love-making.'

Erectile dysfunction (ED, impotence) is defined as a consistent or recurrent inability to attain and/or sustain an erection sufficient for mutually satisfactory sexual intercourse. Many people, including some physicians, believe that erections in the human male are an 'all or none' phenomenon, i.e. that a man who is considered potent usually has a 100 per cent erection and, by contrast, that an 'impotent' man has no erection whatsoever. This is very wrong. Erectile dysfunction does not necessarily mean that there is a total absence of erection. Usually, there is only a partial loss in rigidity. Many men can function sexually even with a twenty to twenty-five per cent impairment in rigidity; that is, with an erection which is just seventy to seventy-five per cent of normal. However, though such an erection will be adequate for sexual intercourse with a woman whose vagina is accustomed to intercourse, it might not be adequate, for example, to penetrate a virginal hymen. I have, in my career, seen many instances where young men who go into matrimony armed with pre-marital sexual experience come to me soon after the wedding with their marriages unconsummated. All their earlier sexual experience has been with women who've had sex before, including commercial sex workers, but all their brides were virgins. These men, so confident and proud of their sexual prowess before marriage, are usually quite aghast that this happened to them, and cannot understand why. Since it is possible nowadays with the help of sophisticated machines to actually measure men's erections, I am able to convincingly and objectively demonstrate to them whether their erections are adequate or not. Doing so without proper evidence would have been unscientific, arbitrary, and suspect. All these young men have now been treated successfully and are leading normal lives.

So, you see, the spectrum of erectile dysfunction is a wide one, with different kinds of presentations at different ages, and multiple causes. The good news is that nearly all causes are treatable successfully nowadays. We'll be talking more about all these in subsequent pages.

And, if you're dying to know the latest on Mr Maggi, yes, he called the other day just to say hello. The first thing he told me was that he is not Mr Maggi any more. I was happy for him. I then asked him if his wife still screams at him. 'Yes, of course, doc,' he said. 'That will never change. The only difference is that nowadays these have become screams of joy, thanks to that magical implant you have inserted. We are very happy now, doc. Thanks very much for everything.'

I smiled to myself. I had created my first crispy noodle.

Take Home Message:

Impotence or erectile dysfunction (ED) is very common. Most ED is usually partial rather than total. Chronic impotence is more often physical than psychological. Many diseases, most notably diabetes and high blood pressure, can cause impotence (see Table I in Appendix). With the world's highest population, and the world's highest prevalence of both diabetes and heart disease, India is arguably the impotence capital of the world. Diagnosis of impotence is made by proper tests, not by guesswork (see Table II in Appendix). Most cases are curable (see Table III in Appendix). Proper specialist consultation is recommended for the diagnosis and management of ED. Quacks and dubious 'aphrodisiacs' can be dangerous.

For further information on erectile dysfunction (ED, impotence), the interested reader is referred to *http://www.andrology.com* and *http://www.impotency.co.in*

2

Fallacies about Phalluses

There is this particularly pestilent yellow car duster vendor at the traffic light near my office, who just doesn't take 'no' for an answer. For days on end, I've watched quietly from the rear seat while he has harangued my driver with his spiel, '*Khareed lo saab. Sirph dus rupiya saab. Bahut badaa size hai saab! (Please buy it sir. Only ten rupees sir ! Very large size sir!)*' My driver would politely say, '*Nahin chaahiye,*' every time, but to no avail. '*Bahut badaa size hai saab! Bahut badaa size hai saab!*' he'd go on. This went on day after day, for months. Then, one day, I lost it completely and couldn't take it any more. I decided to teach this guy a lesson.

My driver and I hatched a conspiracy. So, the next time this vendor accosted us with his pitch and started rubbing his dusters on our windscreen, my driver winked lewdly at him and said, '*Nahin chahiye mujhe. Mera tumhare se bhi bahut badaa hai! Dikhaoon kya? (I don't want it. Mine's much larger than even yours! Shall I show you?!)*'

The double entendre did it. The vendor looked poleaxed for a moment and then vanished like lightning. He never came towards our car ever again. My driver still sports a smug grin whenever we pass that traffic light.

Mere suggestion of penis size seems to have a petrifying effect on most men. One doesn't see men squirming at Arnold Schwarzenegger's muscles, Albert Einstein's brains, or Bill Gates' bank balance, but just tell a man that yours is bigger than his and he's completely crushed. *Show* him it's bigger and he's finished! You might have noticed this phenomenon at public toilets; how guys will go to great, acrobatic lengths to ensure that you can't lean over and take a peek at their unmentionables. They don't want to allow you that size power over them.

When it comes to human penis size, it appears that size is everything, and that bigger is better. Even well-stacked guys won't mind a bit extra. The situation is quite analogous to the hang-ups women have about breast size. Yet, some very busty women will go in for aesthetic breast reduction surgery (remember Katy Mirza?), but the man with the anaconda between his legs already will still want a bit more.

The obsession with penis size is as old as the human race, and possibly even pre-dates it. If you've ever observed chimpanzees and gorillas at zoos, you'll have noticed that they are quite involved with their penises too, but they don't spend their lives monomaniacally obsessing about penis size like humans do.

It is amazing how meticulously some of my patients have studied their penises. One young man had actually taken weekly measurements of his penis over a two-year period. He had scrupulously maintained a chart, which he proudly showed me. It was almost like he was expecting his penis to grow or something. I wondered if he had any other occupation and whether he measured his penis in his office too. I wanted to give him a job in my office. Lots of penises of all kinds here. The chap would probably need to put in a lot of overtime.

And then there was this other chap who rattled off all his penile measurements: length, circumference and girth, in double decimal figures. I was quite certain that he had used vernier scales.

Why are men so fixated about penis size? Does it really make such a big difference?

Here are the facts:

The largest human penis ever reported is eighteen inches long and six inches in circumference. Do I see you squirming with envy? Don't. Such guys don't have it good at all, like you might imagine. It has been shown that such penises are at severe mechanical disadvantage in the erect state and are at high risk of developing erectile dysfunction (impotence) and sustaining fractures.

Of course, there is certainly something like a basic penis size. A basic flaccid penis size, and a basic erect penis size. The former is important if you live in a nudist colony, are a professional stripper, or a flasher in club locker rooms or local trains. The latter is important in the bedroom, or wherever is your preferred location for sex, and if you are a porn star. Flaccid penis length has no direct correlation with erect penile length. Smaller penises are known to enlarge more during erection than those penises that are large in the flaccid state.

Yes, yes, I know you are dying to know what the average measurements for humans are, and that you even have a ruler handy to check out where you stand. But before I tell you that, I'd like to warn you that any information you might have obtained from penis enlargement or lengthening sites, or from websites that advertise aphrodisiacs and other dubious sex remedies, is very likely to be misleading. These are sites that peddle all kinds of cures for small penises: surgery, pills, and devices called penis extenders. It is in the business interest of these sites to artificially inflate the figures for 'average' human penis size, and make most guys feel inadequate. Also, many of the penis size surveys are self-reported surveys, i.e. patients send in their own penis measurements. It has been found that such surveys always report higher averages than those studies that are conducted in a hospital setting where the measurements are obtained by technical personnel. Men, it appears, are notorious liars when it comes to reporting their own penis size.

Here are a few reliable studies from the international literature that I consider important. These should mitigate some of your concerns about penis size.

A medical study conducted by Wessells *et al* at the University of California at San Francisco, which was published in the *Journal of Urology* in 1996, found that average flaccid penile length was 8.8 cm (3.5 inches) and that average erect penile length was 12.9 cm (just over five inches). This was a multi-racial study. Another medical study conducted in the Philippines, and published in the *International Journal of Impotence Research* (2003), found that the average erect penile length was 12.1 cm for orientals and 12.9 cm for occidentals. A Brazilian and a German medical study reported slightly longer erect penises (5.7 inches erect). Condom manufacturers Ansell, makers of *Lifestyles* condoms, who are keen to make condoms for all penis sizes in order to reduce condom failure, found that seventy-five per cent of penises have an erect length of between 4.5 inches and 5.5 inches. In general, the average penis size of blacks is slightly larger than of whites, is slightly larger than in Asians.

Then, there is the issue of 'satisfying' a woman. Many men are unsure if they are — or will be — able to do this and whether penis size is an issue here at all. Most believe it is, but this is only somewhat true. Very short and/or very slender penises are certainly a problem. If a lady has to ask, 'Are you in?', it is definitely a major fiasco. In most other cases, the walls of the vaginal entrance, being elastic, will close snugly around the penis during coitus. It is only the first two inches of the vagina that are actually sensitive to erogenous stimuli. Thus, the average penis should be perfectly capable of delivering the goods, and if the lady is dissatisfied, the cause must lie elsewhere than in the size of the penis. Also, contrary to popular belief, women are not so fixated on penis size. Studies have shown that only about fifteen per cent of women think that size is very important. To the woman, it is the performance that matters most.

Nearly fifty-four per cent of men feel that their penis is small. In most cases, this fear is probably unfounded.

This perhaps explains why I get several requests to perform penis enlargement surgery every week. This subject is a vast one, and a detailed discussion is outside the purview of this book. Nonetheless, it is important to state a few things here. There is a lot of misleading information out there on this subject, and many fall victims to the lure of dangerous hype. I have seen many men with maimed and disfigured penises following unscrupulous enlargement surgery, which they did not even require in the first place.

When it comes to penis enlargement surgery, I classify my patients into two groups — the 'needy' and the 'greedy'. The needy are those with penises that are smaller *than the lower limit of the average range.* This smallness can be due to congenital (from birth) causes or could be secondary to other local conditions. These patients really require — and can use — enlargement surgery. The greedy are those who are adequately endowed but nothing will convince them of this fact. I dissuade most such from undergoing enlargement surgery. However, sometimes, untreated, these patients may have so many psychosexual and self-esteem problems that it is best to accede to their request and give them the few inches they so desperately crave. After all, if a woman can augment her breasts, why can't a man augment his penis? However, it must be emphasised that this surgery is still controversial and must be performed only judiciously by experienced surgeons at reputed centres.

Remember, the human penis is not always like an Onida TV set. The neighbour's envy may not be the owner's pride if the operation has been botched.

For further information on penis lengthening and girth enhancement, the interested reader is referred to *http://www.andrology.com/penisaugmentation.htm*

3

The Computerisation of Manhood

Over the past few years, there has been a massive influx of IT (Information Technology) guys into southern Indian cities, from both within and outside of India. It is inevitable, therefore, that one bumps into them sooner or later. The following happened to me once.

I was sitting with this bunch of IT gasbags. Supercilious, bright, young men — in their late twenties and mid-thirties, at the most. At forty, I was already a living fossil as far as they were concerned. Naturally, they were doing all the talking, and I was doing the listening. When IT guys talk, you have no choice. There's no chance of getting in a word edgeways. So, I was just nodding along dumbly for a while, and then gave up altogether. They were all talking about the incredible shape of things to come, all thanks to IT. These guys made telemedicine and robotic surgery seem like pedestrian stuff. Also, I was going dizzy trying to figure out how many zeroes there are in a million and a billion. I still don't know. In my field, we generally associate these numbers only with the population figures of Indian cities and the nation, respectively.

Finally, one of the kinder ones noticed my physical presence. He turned to me and asked condescendingly, 'Hey doc! What does IT mean to you, huh?'

For a while, I thought that it might be a good idea to act dumb. They thought I was daft anyway. 'Intercourse Techniques,' 'Impotence Treatment,' and 'Income Tax' all came to mind. But I desisted. It is dangerous to surrender to bullies.

Instead, I said, 'Actually, we have IT applications in andrology, too. We convert software to hardware.'

I thought I saw the windbags looking at me with new respect.

'Geez! No kidding, doc?' said one of the whiz kids who had just returned from the US of A and sported an accent thicker than a fourth generation Southerner's. 'How the hell do you do that, ma'an? I mean, transform software to hardware! Never heard of it.'

I figured that he was already conjuring up visions of his next billion, extrapolating from my idea. All of a sudden, I felt very important. I took a deep breath, sat erect, straightened my back, and slid forward in my seat. I was not going to give up this table-turning opportunity easily. I had never expected these helium balloons to ever hand the mike to me. Now that I had the chance to speak, I decided to teach them a proper lesson. I cleared my throat pompously and began venting pure spleen.

'Well, you see, in my specialty, I see many men with impotence, also known as erectile dysfunction or ED'. I could see a few creased brows and some puzzled stares. These guys were impatient; I quickly continued, 'Men with ED come to me with wares that were once hard, but have now become soft. After I treat them, their software gets converted to hardware,' I concluded dramatically.

This was just the first jab. I then proceeded to deliver my knockout punch. 'We even have computers to diagnose impotence nowadays. I can apply a machine on a man's penis, here in Hyderabad, and his girlfriend can monitor his erections online in Nebraska even. The machine can tell whether one is man enough or not. If you don't believe me, you can have yourself checked out on my machines for free and see for yourself,' I offered charitably.

All of a sudden, the balloons looked punctured. My day was made! Deflating these dirigibles is great fun, I concluded.

Spurred by the taste of first blood, I proceeded to hammer more and more nails into their coffins. I embarked on a one-hour soliloquy on the Rigiscan® machine and various other tests for impotence. No one dared interrupt me. They were all mortified that I might computerise their manhood and unravel dark secrets for all to see. The macho men had suddenly turned into pansies.

Not long ago, the diagnosis of impotence was made either by the patient himself, or by his partner. The visit to the 'doctor', if it ever happened, was purely for treatment. It was a foregone conclusion that the problems were all 'in the mind'; in other words, psychological. If not that, the chap was purportedly paying the price for having masturbated excessively or something. Nobody ever examined him or tested him. Patients sat fully clothed in front of their physicians. The doctor didn't even check if the man had a penis at all. Such was the state of affairs.

Imagine being told that you have a hernia, or piles, without being asked to drop your pants. Or being told that a weakness in your arm, which you fear might be the beginnings of a stroke, is all only 'in the mind', without any kind of workup*. Unthinkable, isn't it? Yet, when it came to men's andrological complaints, this is what always happened. Until recently, everyone was living in darkness on this subject. That such things happen even today, at many places, is a different story.

Then, in 1982, a new era in andrology was born when Frenchman Ronald Virag induced an erection in his office by injecting a drug called papaverine into a man's penis. This was the first time in medical history that it became possible for an erection to be induced and measured in a clinical setting. Subjective descriptions of erections were out. Objective measurements were introduced. Injecting a standard dose of a drug into the penis, and checking if the resulting erectile response was rigid enough, became the first ever method of objectively studying erectile dysfunction.

At about the same time, a physician named Karacan, in Houston, Texas, began measuring human erectile activity during sleep. It was long known that human beings develop erections during sleep**. These erections occur during the REM

---

*A thorough medical examination, including laboratory tests, x-ray, etc.

**This is nothing to be proud of. Primate monkeys develop them too!

(Rapid Eye Movement), dream phase of sleep. Except in a few situations, these erections are considered truly representative of a man's erectile ability since they are bereft of the anxiety components that accompany the waking state. Karacan invented a NPT (Nocturnal Penile Tumescence) device. This was a groundbreaking machine, but it failed to measure the all-important parameter of erection, *viz.* rigidity. The invention of the Rigiscan® machine soon thereafter solved this problem.

The IT balloons were listening intently. I told them more about doppler and ultrasound studies to image and measure flow in the penile arteries, about dynamic infusion cavernosometric studies to evaluate the penile veins, about plethysmography, electromyography, phalloarteriography...I was having fun.

The message seemed to have gotten across. Shoulders were stooped now. The 'Southerner' asked me, 'Tell me doc, how does a man know if he is rigid enough, and whether he is lasting long enough, and that his wife isn't unhappy and faking it? That he isn't deluding himself about his manhood?'

Even so many years ago, I was simply too seasoned to fall for this ploy. I've encountered just too many guys trying to ask what seems like a general interest question but is actually their personal andrological problem in decoy mode. No, it wasn't going to work with me.

'Six thirty p.m. next Friday, at my office, is a good time and place to discuss this,' I said. 'Call my secretary and confirm your appointment, please.'

Touché!

I walked away whistling a tune from _The Good, the Bad and the Ugly_. In my mind, there was this image that I was Clint Eastwood, blowing the smoke off the tip of my just-fired gun. How dare anybody think me a fossil?!

Take Home Message:

Many sophisticated tests are available today for the diagnosis and objective evaluation of impotence (erectile dysfunction, ED) should the need arise (see Table II in Appendix). These tests help differentiate psychological from physical impotence, and measure its severity. They are useful not only in day-to-day andrological practice, but are also very valuable in courts of law, when divorce has been filed for on grounds of impotence. Not only can these tests confirm impotence, they can also protect the falsely accused by proving potency. For information about these tests, check out _http://www.AndromedaAndrologyCenter.com_

4

Men Can Be Curvaceous Too

Adoctor's office is not exactly a place where you'd expect people to walk in with a smile, whistling away. People are more likely to look downcast and miserable. Ergo, I have seen many Sad Sacks over the years. But this particular newlywed young man, whom I saw some time ago, really took the cake. When I saw him, even I felt like crying. Such was his impact.

Mr Lacrimose (Lacri, for short) entered my office hurriedly when announced, and sat down in front of me without much preamble. 'Docky,' he began twitchily, 'My marriage is on the rocks. My wife thinks I don't love her. I love her like nobody's business, but she just doesn't believe me. Nothing can convince her. I don't want to live, docky. I want to end my life. You are my last hope.'

That sounded ominous. I love challenges, but taking on something like this seemed a bit daunting, even to a man with my experience. I fixed my gaze empathetically on Lacri and asked him, 'What makes you say all this? Things in the first six months of marriage ought to be hunky-dory.' The tragedy usually begins a bit later, I wanted to tell him, but I desisted, thinking that his already swollen tear glands might rupture.

'I don't know how to tell you, docky. It's all so embarrassing and complicated. There's this girl next door whom I used to like, before marriage, but somehow things never worked out between us. My wife, who knows about this, thinks that I still love that girl and that's why I have not been able to consummate my marriage even after six long months.'

'But is that the real reason?', I ferreted.

'Not at all, doc,' said Mr Lacrimose, 'I've gotten over that girl completely. But my wife is convinced that she's the reason. You see, every time I try to make love to my wife, my penis points ninety degrees away from her, and she thinks that it is pointing towards the bedroom of the girl next door,' he finished miserably.

I told him to relax and not to worry and that his wife, having read too many Mills and Boon and Barbara Cartland novels, probably still believed in the magnetic attraction theory. 'Have you ever tried to explain to your wife that such magnetism is purely metaphorical, and that the human penis is a non-magnetic object?', I proffered helpfully.

'You try explaining to her, doc. I've tried everything, and nothing seems to work. I've got cricks in my neck, back and hips, trying to perform bedroom acrobatics. Once I nearly broke my penis even. But she just doesn't understand.'

Hmmm...this lady certainly has a clear sense of direction and purpose, and likes to get straight to the point, I surmised. Too bad that Lacri was missing the point every time. It now became clear to me that I had to take his matter in my own hands and straighten it out. I decided also to give him another sobriquet. Bentdick seemed like a good second name.

Mr Lacrimose Bentdick, it turned out, suffered from a condition known as a congenital penile curvature. A simple operation straightened out matters completely, and the couple is now busy making up for lost time. LB, in fact, told me recently that his wife is now complaining that he loves her too much, and asked whether I could do something about this now.

Some people are truly hard to please.

Curves and bends of the penis are common and affect fifteen per cent of all men. Penile curvature can be congenital (present from birth) or acquired (developed later in life). It may or may not be associated with other anomalies. In isolated penile curvature, there is only a bend, without any associated abnormalities. The penis may curve or deviate upward, downward, or to the side. The deformity usually becomes most pronounced in the erect state. The penis often appears normal in the flaccid (non-erect) state. Sometimes, there is an additional component of twist, or torsion. Curves, bends, and twists can all co-exist in the same penis. Men with isolated penile curvature usually have no problems with their erectile rigidity. Also, in most cases the curvature is mild and does not interfere with sexual activity. Such curvatures can be left alone, untreated. All that the patient will require is some reassurance.

In some cases, however, the curvature is serious. This can make intercourse difficult or even impossible. In addition to pure deformity, additionally, there may be severe cosmetic disfigurement in the erect state. In my practice, over the past two decades, I have seen some penises with a ninety-degree deformity even, meaning the penis really looks like a right angle. And then there are some others who develop serious psychosexual disturbances as a consequence of the curvature. About twenty to thirty per cent of patients with penile curvature will eventually require surgery for one or more of these reasons. The operation is safe and gives excellent cosmetic and functional results, if done by the right hands, without jeopardising sexual function.

In acquired penile curvature, there is usually a contributory cause. This cause superimposes itself on a previously normal penis and causes deformity. In such cases, secondary impotence is not uncommon, and sexual intercourse is sometimes impossible. The commonest cause of an acquired penile curvature is the condition known as Peyronie's disease. Named after François Gigot de La Peyronie, surgeon to King Louis XV of France, this is a condition where a lump or nodule develops in the penile shaft. Pain is a concomitant in the early stages, and a progressive deformity develops over the next several months. Peyronie's disease usually affects the elderly. Surgery is indicated if the deformity precludes sexual intercourse, causes impotence (erectile dysfunction), or induces serious psychosexual disturbance. In recent years, Peyronie's disease has been made famous by former US president, Bill Clinton, who suffered from the disease.

There are many operations available for Peyronie's disease. Some are popular, yet ineffective, and *vice versa*. Many have become obsolete. My personal preference is for the operation described by me. This fetched me the coveted Herbert Newman* international award some years ago. Known as the 'penile dermal flap operation' or the 'Krishnamurti' operation, this is a simple, ingenious operation that uses locally available penile skin to straighten the penis and cure deformity. Results are excellent. Patients with Peyronie's disease who have superadded impotence (erectile dysfunction, ED) will require additional treatment. Those whose impotence does not respond to conservative measures will eventually require the surgical insertion of penile prostheses. There are some other causes of bends and curves too. The approach to these is pretty similar.

All in all, curves of the penis are just a straightforward twist.

> *There was this man from Tashkent*
> *Whose apparatus, it appears, was very bent*
> *He tried, and he tried*
> *And his wife often cried*
> *Because, instead of coming, he went !*

Now you know that men can sometimes drive women crazy with their curves too.

Retributive justice, I suppose?

---

*The highest international award for original clinical research in the field of impotence

Take Home Message:

Deformities of the penis are not uncommon, and occur in varying degrees. The deformity may or may not be associated with other abnormalities. Some deformities are present from birth. These are called congenital curvatures. Others come on later and are called acquired curvatures. Peyronie's disease is a classical example of the latter. Minor degrees of curvature and deformity may not cause any serious handicap, physical or psychological. These can be left untreated. Severe deformity, impotence and psychosexual issues may necessitate surgery. When performed at centres of excellence, surgery provides very good results.

Further information on penile curvatures and Peyronie's disease can be obtained on *http://www.PeyroniesDisease.org*

5

Azhar Faces ED!

Newspapers have become needlessly complex nowadays. Not only does every home receive several newspapers, each one is thicker than its rivals and countless supplements and booklets keep falling out. One doesn't know where to start, what to read. Gone are the good old days when there was only one slim newspaper per home, and one could grab all the news in just a few minutes. Today, reading the newspapers comprehensively every morning is a luxury that only a few can afford.

Scanning all the headlines once from back to front, and then reading the newspapers in detail and digesting them as one is getting rid of the undigested, is the only comprehensive way for me. On one morning, some years ago, I did not have this luxury, and had to be content with just a cursory headlines scan. In a little while, I was due to deliver a lecture on ED (erectile dysfunction, impotence) to a bunch of doctors, and I didn't want to be late. Just as the driver announced that the car was ready, my eyes chanced upon a front page headline that screamed 'Azhar Faces ED'*.

There was no time for details. I had to rush.

It was a very disturbed ride to the conference venue for me. I just could not apply my mind to the lecture I was due to deliver soon. 'How can it be?!', I wondered, too shocked for words. Not so long ago, I had heard cricket greats say that despite being the oldest player in the Indian team, Azhar was perhaps the fittest and most agile of them all. How then, could he be facing ED? Physical fitness, in fact, is said to protect a person from facing ED. Besides, I wondered, how can such an embarrassing and personal problem make front page headlines? Do these reporters have no sense of decency, prying into the bedrooms of our poor celebs? I was angry, and curious. Even in a country like the USA, only three to seven per cent of men facing ED admit to the problem and seek medical help for it. In fact, seventy-four per cent of men in the US cite embarrassment as the number one reason for why they don't see a doctor. In a conservative country like India, these figures must be worse. I thought that it was pretty bold of Azhar to want to belong among the minority yet again. He had already played the minority card once.

Besides, hadn't Azhar only recently taken a second wife? And had a child? Or was I making a mistake? He wouldn't have

---

*This headline appeared some years ago, and that was when this essay of mine was first written, albeit in a different form. The reader is advised to keep that time frame in context while reading this piece.

been able to do all that if he was facing ED, I thought to myself. Furthermore, to my knowledge, he had no underlying health condition that would predispose him to facing ED. If he had had any, the whole world would have known. The greedy corporates would have used his illness to market their products, and the media would have gone berserk speculating. So, an underlying illness was ruled out. Then what was it?

I was really upset, and concerned. Naturally. Azhar was every Hyderabadi's favourite cricketer. My mind wouldn't stop worrying. The lecture is a minor issue, I told myself. I've spoken on the same subject so many times before that I can deliver this talk even in my sleep, I rationalised. I was convinced that this other matter was much more serious. Since it involves not just cricket but a cricket captain too, I believed that this must be rated a national calamity. After all, in India, cricketers' privates are also public.

It is true that ten per cent of men face ED and that the figure rises to a staggering fifty-two per cent for men above forty. But wasn't Azhar on the right side of forty? I knew he was. Could this mean that he was among the unfortunate ten per cent in the under-forty age group who faced ED? Terrible, terrible, I thought to myself. But this was no time for melodrama. As a responsible pioneer in my field, I had to take the initiative in solving this problem.

My first considerations were patriotic. Will Azhar seek the help of some American or other specialist for his condition? I knew that it was fashionable for our celebs to fly out even for coughs and colds, but I didn't want Azhar to waste his money.

I didn't want the national exchequer to spend lakhs of rupees flying in an andrological Chittaranjan Ranawat either. It is bad enough that we have brain drains and many other kinds of drains in our country. No point in adding an andrological drain, I decided.

I wanted to treat Azhar for free, and conserve valuable foreign exchange. On second thoughts, I revised that decision, and thought that one of Azhar's Armani jackets would be fair fee for my services. I particularly liked his beige one. I had seen him with that one on in a society/fashion glossy recently. I desperately wanted to lose weight and be able to fit into that. I thought I'd look pretty handsome in it too.

'What the heck? India is andrologically self-sufficient,' I screamed aloud in the back seat of my car. My driver, who has seen me in my looney moods on many earlier occasions, didn't bat an eyelid. He glanced cursorily at the rearview mirror, rolled his eyeballs skywards once, and drove on.

'Was Azhar a cyclist?', I wondered. Hah, that was probably it! Many fitness afficionados use bicycles. And bicycles can make men face ED. It appears that the seats of most conventional bicycles cause friction injuries to the rider's perineum — the portion of the anatomy between the scrotum and the anus. The arteries to the penis have to traverse this region in order to carry blood to it. Chronic bicycle riding can damage these arteries and cause men to face ED.

If bikes were the culprits, then Azhar might require a microsurgical bypass operation, I thought. I quickly rehearsed the steps of the operation in my mind. I had done the first one of its kind in India** many years ago. I'd better not goof it up this time. These operative steps would come in handy even if the ED was caused by a hit to the pelvis or perineum. Hits to the unmentionables are after all an occupational hazard for cricketers and another important reason for facing ED. Or had Azhar developed a spinal problem? That was another culprit we needed to rule out. Spine injuries are very common in sport.

What else? What else?!

My andrological peregrinations were rudely interrupted by the car pulling to a halt outside the convention centre where my conference was being conducted. Couldn't the organisers have scheduled this stupid lecture on another day? There are so many more important things happening in my field in the country today. I swore under my breath and walked in.

I requested the chairman to keep the day's newspapers handy for my perusal right after my talk, and went through the motions of the lecture. Though this was some small compensation for my abbreviated motions that morning, it still didn't take my mind off the former Indian cricket captain. I finally requested an expediting of the valedictories and nose-dived for the nearest newspaper.

**The first microsurgical revascularisation (bypass) operation for impotence in India was performed by me on 2 January 1991, on a twenty-one-year old man who had become impotent following a pelvic fracture sustained in a vehicular accident.

To my horror, it turned out that ED stood for 'Enforcement Directorate'! There goes my beige Armani jacket, I thought, but felt happy for Azhar nonetheless. The medical brand of ED is one woe he doesn't need right now.

Take Home Message:

Many men are at risk of developing erectile dysfunction but do not know it. Some of these ED risk factors are outlined in http://www.andrology.com/EDriskfactors.htm. Awareness of these conditions can help a person take timely preventive / curative action. More importantly, such awareness can help to connect the ED to the underlying risk factor. This causal relationship is often missed by both physician and patient because of ignorance. More than eighty per cent of chronic erectile dysfunction is caused by physical, or organic, problems, rather than by psychological, or functional ones, as is generally supposed.

Thus, more chronic impotence results from causes 'between the legs' than from causes 'between the ears'. Beware of false propaganda by irresponsible physicians to the contrary.

6

The Vas Deferens between Men and Women

This is about the young couple that came to see me some years ago for a family planning consultation. The couple had two children, but looked like that was one too many already. Since they couldn't do much about the children they already had, they were determined not to have a third at any cost, I supposed. Their determination showed, especially on the wife's face. Apparently, the lady's obstetrician had tried to persuade her to undergo a tubal ligation (female sterilisation) operation, but the lady had refused. Instead, she wanted her husband to undergo a vasectomy. They were in my office to check out the pros and cons of a vasectomy operation.

It seemed to me that I was not really necessary here. The couple looked like they were ready to sterilise each other right then and there without my assistance, given half a chance and a quarter of a scalpel. They might have even done so, were it not for Munna, their obnoxious, two-year-old brat. This nuisance was sequentially plucking at the stationery on my desk, his mother's salwar (loose pants worn with long shirts), and his dad's spectacles, in no particular order, with a manic kind of gusto. For respite, he ran around the entire office, fancying himself to be a whistling express train.

Under such circumstances, it was understandably hard for Munna's parents to perform surgery on one another. Injuries could occur and the wrong body parts might get cut off.

I had to finally silence Munna the Pest with a killer look and the flashing of a fifty ml syringe with a huge attached needle. For those who might not know, the combined length of this syringe–needle contraption is about the length of a grown man's forearm. Once Munna saw that, he abruptly sat down in a corner, like a frozen bar of ice cream, for the remainder of the afternoon. I shuddered to imagine what his sibling must be like. It was no wonder that the poor parents wanted sterilisation.

'Doctor,' the wife began, 'We want to know about vasectomy.'

'I can talk for several hours on the topic but I guess you might not have that much time or interest. What exactly do you want to know?', I offered, as efficiently as I could.

'Doctor, I feel that it is much easier for him to undergo a vasectomy than for me to go through a tubal ligation. Why must it be me all the time? I've already gone through two Caesarean sections. He's such a hypocrite. He tells everybody that he's the new millennium man, but deep inside he is nothing but a Male Chauvinist Pig. He does not want to undergo the operation and he's trying to turn the tables on me with all kinds of excuses. Please explain to him. Plea...sss..e.'

I turned to Mr Touch-Me-Not and asked him what his reservations about vasectomy were.

'Well, doctor, I've heard horrid things about the operation,' he said.

'That was only during the days of the Emergency. Times have changed,' I said, soothingly.

'No, no, doctor. That's not what he means. He thinks that a vasectomy causes all kinds of weaknesses. Please explain to him that it does not,' Ms Sterilise Him commanded.

This young mother of two certainly knows a thing or two about vasectomised men, I thought to myself, but, being a good doctor, I dismissed the thought and resisted pondering how. That was outside the purview of this consultation; and none of my business anyway.

Since the gamut of imagined weaknesses that could be caused by a vasectomy range from 'total body weakness' to 'sudden death', I thought that it might be simpler for Mr Touch-Me-Not to indicate to me what his specific apprehensions were. I told him so.

'Well, I've heard that a vasectomy operation causes impotence, stops ejaculation, and induces many kinds of weaknesses,' he said lamely, shiftily avoiding any eye contact whilst speaking. 'Besides, the part is sooooo...so...delicate. I can't bear to have any incisions made on it, doc. How will I walk? How will I ever have sex again? Oooooo! I shudder at the mere prospect. Do you give general anaesthesia for such major operations? Will you keep me in hospital for a week?', he was eager to know.

Amused? I don't find it funny at all.

I see many such men. All of them think that their wives have pachyderm hide in the place of skin, and that these women don't feel any pain at all during labour, Caesarean sections, and several other operations that women undergo from time to time. What two-faced, sissy hypocrites these men are! It is sad, but true, that most Indian men are like this. It must have something to do with the *khandaan-ka-chiraag* (light of the family), *laadla-beta* (darling son) syndrome that is so glamourised on Indian celluloid. Anyone who has seen a fifty plus on-screen Dharmendra run into Nirupa Roy's arms shouting 'Maaaaa!' will know exactly what I am talking about. Mr Touch-Me-Not was of that same mollycoddle ilk. No doubt about it.

'Have you ever known anyone who has become impotent or has developed ejaculatory problems after vasectomy?', I asked him.

Once again, he glanced evasively all over the room, taking his time to answer. Finally, he shook his head.

'Then who told you all this rubbish?', I asked.

'My friends told me,' said Mr Touch-me-Not. When I asked him if these friends had themselves undergone vasectomies, he said that they hadn't, and that such potential complications were the very reasons why. To avoid such 'extremely injurious' side effects, all these friends had subjected their wives to a tubal ligation instead! These poor wives actually believed their husbands, and not wanting them to suffer such 'life-threatening' side effects, these meek ladies submitted themselves to the gynaecologist's scalpel.

It was a heinous national conspiracy.

I was determined to do something about this. I spoke for the next several minutes, explaining the facts as they are, allaying apprehensions, and placing matters in correct perspective. Luckily for both him and me, Mr Touch-Me-Not was very receptive.

I began by telling them that the vas deferens is the tube that carries sperm from the testis up into the pelvis. Here, the sperm join the seminal secretions from other glands and get expelled in the ejaculate. Sperms in the semen are responsible for fertilisation of the egg. A vasectomy is an operation in which the vas deferens is cut and tied off. This blocks the sperm from entering the ejaculate and thus sterilises the male.

A vasectomy is usually performed under local anaesthesia. It takes just a few minutes and the patient usually goes back home or to the office within a few hours. It is a very safe operation and carries a very high success rate. The vasa deferentia (plural for vas deferens) are located in the scrotum. Thus, they are practically outside the body and hence, easily accessible. They are also just a few millimetres below the skin. By contrast, the Fallopian tubes in the female are located deep in the pelvic cavity, right inside the body. The complications of a tubectomy are thus potentially a lot more serious than those of a vasectomy.

Also, should the need arise, a vasectomy can be much more successfully reversed than a tubectomy, using modern microsurgical methods. I perform several of these operations regularly, with very good results. In fact, nowadays, due to a rise in medical tourism, I increasingly perform these on patients coming in from other countries too.

The vas deferens has no anatomical or physiological connection with the penis, though the two are *juxtaposed*. Hence, it is impossible for a vasectomy operation to cause any impotence or sexual dysfunction, and any perceived weaknesses after operation are purely imaginary, and just a big, convenient myth. Similarly, ejaculatory function is not affected either, since the ejaculatory apparatus is located much higher up, in the pelvis. Also, a vasectomy results in only a ten to twenty per cent reduction in the total semen volume, because most of the seminal fluid is secreted by the seminal vesicles and the prostate gland, which are located much higher up in the pelvis and are not even touched during a vasectomy.

'So, you see, in short, a vasectomy is a very safe and successful, minimally invasive operation that is performed under local anaesthesia, and allows you to go home in a few hours. It has no serious adverse effects,' I concluded pedantically.

Mr Touch-Me-Not looked like he was about to weep. He rose from his chair, walked to his wife and put his arms around her. 'I'm sorry, really, really sorry darling,' he said, his voice choking with emotion. 'I am sorry if I have hurt you. I was really misinformed.'

He wiped his tear-drenched face with his shirt sleeve and turned to me, 'Can we fix up the operation for tomorrow itself, doc ?', he asked, still stifling his sobs.

My gaze fell on Munna. Suddenly, a warning bell went off in my head. 'We can even do it right now,' I enthused. 'It'll take only a few minutes.'

I'd have done anything to prevent another Munna from happening.

Take Home Message:

A vasectomy, or a male sterilisation operation, is a very simple, safe and effective procedure. It carries very high success rates and low complication rates. It is much simpler to perform than a female sterilisation operation, and is easier to reverse, should the need arise. Reversal also carries higher success rates, especially if performed at centres of microsurgical excellence. It is wrong to suppose that a vasectomy causes many fearsome complications and side effects. It does not.

Thus, unless there are specific reasons against it, a vasectomy should unhesitatingly be the sterilisation procedure of choice for couples. Check out *http://www.IndiaInfertility.com* or *http://www.AndromedaAndrologyCenter.com*.

7

Troglodytes and Gentlemen

Human sexuality is a very complex subject. In clinical practice, one sees distinctly different cases and fresh twists every day, and there is no singular algorithm for all situations. Treatment programmes have to be custom made every time. No matter how long one has been in the business, it is impossible to have seen it all and to have done it all. Every day is a new learning experience. The following case history should illustrate my point.

Recently, a newlywed couple came to see me. They had been married for just five days. Their problem? Yup, you've guessed it! Their problem was that they hadn't 'done it' yet. Five nights together, but no sexual intercourse. Seven people trooped into my office at the allotted appointment time: the couple, three people from the girl's side, and two from the boy's! I craned my neck to peer over their shoulders and check whether there were any more. Anything is possible in our populous country.

People who walk into my office will notice at once that it is a small place, and that I have seating only for two people other than myself. This arrangement, of course, is deliberate, and is intended to provide privacy to my patients. The gang of seven noticed this configuration as soon as it entered. Yet, no one took the hint. They all stayed put inside the room. Ostensibly, the sex life of this couple was the business of the entire family. Every one of them, it appeared, wanted a piece of the action. It is not funny how common this is in India.

Such a scenario, of course, is not new to me at all. I have had, in the past, more than twelve people accompanying a couple into my inner office. That motley group had included many village elders and local leaders whose many responsibilities apparently included human coital welfare, in addition to other multitudinous welfare programmes. Hats off to these guys! I marvel quite often at how these chaps can have their fingers simultaneously in so many different pies. One has heard of people being in public life, but this 'being in *pubic* life' aspect was a new one to me. In addition to the army of twelve generals, there were some other 'friends and well-wishers' in the waiting room as well. Those must be the infantrymen, I surmised.

I made eye contact with each member of the coital welfare army individually, and gave every single one of them a wide, beaming smile. And this, for me, is a big effort. I'm normally a grumpy sort of guy. But in this situation, I had a specific motive for such exertion. I wanted to convey to these sex soldiers that my office is a warm, friendly place, where I help people. These guys radiated a belligerence that was not one bit conducive to any kind of peaceable settlement. The 'boy's side' was ready to kill the 'girl's side', and *vice versa*. I shuddered to imagine the effect this might have had on the poor newlyweds, and decided that this killer instinct first needed to be neutralised, if we wished to make any progress.

To state that this endeavour of mine was futile, would be putting it mildly. Nothing changed even after several minutes. The belligerence remained.

I have learnt from experience that one mustn't ever initiate proceedings in such situations. You never know whose sentiments you might inadvertently ignite, just with your innocuous opening line. I waited patiently. Meantime, a lot of heated whispers were being exchanged between the two 'rival factions'. Finally, it seemed that they had arrived at a consensus about who would open the attack.

'*Daaktr saab,*' one of the senior generals finally addressed me, pointing to the new groom, '*Inho to mard ich nahin hain*' (this guy is not a man at all).

I was visibly upset by this elderly man's derogatory language, and decided to stop pussyfooting around any longer. I ordered everyone but the patient out of my office.

I was expecting some resistance to this, and so was not surprised when the wife protested, 'If I leave the room doc, this man will tell you all kinds of lies about me.'

I let her stay. I'm not a one man army that can take on a dozen belligerents.

I spent nearly an hour with them. I spoke to the couple first, and then separately with the husband and the wife. Many interesting facts emerged. First, that the marriage was a totally 'arranged' one. The bride and the groom hadn't even met before the wedding. In keeping with an ancient Indian tradition, they had simply 'okayed' the alliance after seeing passport-sized photographs of the prospective spouses. The match was fixed by elders, pretty much like in Indian cricket. It seemed quite obvious that the maiden had bowled the groom's middle stump over.

The second fact that emerged was that there was a conspicuous absence of any friendship, affection, or love between man and wife. The arrangement seemed more like a sexual contract. The wife expected the man to perform his contractual obligations like an insatiable stud on his wedding night, without the need for any preliminary equation, relationship or intimacy to develop first. This couple didn't talk at all and the wife didn't even let her husband hold hands affectionately. She wasn't interested.

My patient just couldn't have sex under such circumstances. He was a gentle, educated man who wanted to get to know his wife first, and then move on gradually to sex. He had already had premarital sex in an earlier relationship, and was not in a hurry to prove anything to anybody. His wife, *au contraire*, just wanted to lie on her back and have him finish the job. No hugging, no caressing, no foreplay. She confessed to me that this is what her orthodox upbringing had indoctrinated into her, and was unyielding in her stance. If he was man enough, he ought to be able to do it. What was the need for mushy preliminaries? Showing the immediate relatives stained bed sheets was the name of the game. That's how generations of women before her had consummated a marriage. Everything else came much later. She did not see anything wrong in announcing to all and sundry in the family that she had not yet had sex.

Cave woman, it seemed, was not really extinct.

Upon the insistence of both rival factions, I performed a couple of tests on Mr Gentleman. To me, his acquiescence to the tests itself was proof of his virility. Not surprisingly, all his reports were normal.

Despite this, however, his marriage broke. Apparently, the cave woman couldn't wait any longer for sex to happen. It seemed that she was looking more for a burly rapist than for a refined gentleman. She argued with her parents that her friends who had got married before her had done it three or four times per night in the first few days after marriage itself. Those were the kind of macho husbands she was looking for. Her impression of her own husband was that he was a total *namard* (emasculate).

Her parents complied with her command and took her back to their house. Mr Gentleman became a much maligned man in the social circle.

It saddened me to note that many in our society have yet to outgrow this neanderthal concept of marriage. I felt very bad for Mr Gentleman and the fact that I was not able to help him to amicably negotiate the situation. But I knew, deep inside, that he would bounce back soon.

Just as I had hoped, Mr Gentleman visited me again some time after that. This time, he was accompanied by a pleasant young lady. The couple seemed very much in love, and the air was filled with good vibes. It was very obvious that they were sexually happy, too. I too was very happy for them.

As for Ms Cave Woman, there's been no news. She was probably happily married to a strong and silent caveman who spoke only with his club.

Well...different strokes for different folks!

Take Home Message:

The above case history has many messages. This book, however, merely concerns itself with the andrological one. It is wrong to suppose that all men are lustful creatures who can have sexual intercourse with any partner at all under any and all circumstances. Many men cannot. This might make them temporarily 'impotent' even though there is nothing wrong with their erectile mechanism. Men have sensibilities and sensitivities too, and this must be recognised.

8

The Reincarnation of Proud Peter

Some months ago, my secretary announced a long distance call from someone who claimed to be an old friend. 'Hi, howdy Suds?' the strange voice boomed, sounding very familiar. 'I don't know if you will recollect, Sudhakar, but thirty years ago, you and I were in the same class in school. This is DK; a.k.a. Biceps. Class of 1971. Place me!?'

'Oh my God! You're kidding me!' I exclaimed, almost standing up, clutching the phone receiver tight.

'No, no, I'm not kidding, *yaar*. It IS me! Does our old code, Operation Frog, ring a bell somewhere?'

How could I forget!? Biceps and I were notorious for unleashing into biology class every week, several dozen frogs, from tin *dabbas*. The girls would scream and run all over the place, and the boys would try and act macho, even though panic-stricken. But what took the cake was the sight of the biology professor climbing atop his desk and screaming at all of us. He was the most petrified of all!

Not only was Biceps very much in my class thirty years ago, he was also in the same class for many years. Considering that his classmates spanned several batches, I thought that it was quite elephantine of him to remember and trace me. Apparently, he had read an interview of mine with a leading newspaper in the country where he was now living, and had then traced all my numbers through the internet.

I recall him as being quite tall, compared to me. He was also very strong, menacing-looking, and hairy. I remember many occasions on which he was sent back from class to the dorm to shave his beard. I used to be very impressed by such masculinity in my peers those days. I was yet to attain my puberty fully, and spent many hours looking for at least one or two hairs on my face and legs. I wondered how many years Biceps had spent in the same class, bullying the other kids just like he bullied us.

I remember how, one day, I had staged a coup of sorts by offering to do his homework for him every single day. It was just a piece of cake for me and only took me a few minutes, but to him it was invaluable. He never paid any attention to anything in class, and hence learnt nothing. In return for this major favour, I got the protection of Biceps' flexed biceps, much to the annoyance of the others. Nobody monkeyed with me after that. Biceps and I became best friends. Finally, unfortunately, I had to leave school because I passed all my exams in the first attempt and was not allowed to stay in the same class any longer. Biceps stayed back. Must've been for a long time, I'm sure. We stayed in touch for a year or two, but then lost all contact. I suspect that my mom intercepted and destroyed all his letters after a point. They were pure, unadulterated porn.

It was an effort for me to snap out of my mental peregrinations. 'Hey Biceps! How come, all of a sudden?' I finally managed. He sounded impatient. 'Suds, I'm visiting India next week. Are you going to be in town on Thursday? I need to meet you desperately.' I affirmed that I was very much in town on Thursday. We fixed up an appointment for 8 p.m., the last appointment of the day. The plan was to follow the meeting up with drinks and dinner.

'I have to rush now. These morons have just announced the last and final boarding call. I'm glad I was able to talk to you Suds. See ya Thursday.' The line went dead.

Later that evening, at home, I told my wife about Biceps' call, and asked whether women would feel as strongly about sudden appearances of friends from the distant past. She nodded absently in the affirmative. This was nothing for her. She is used to much stranger questions from me. We then discussed plans for Biceps' dinner. I recalled that Biceps used to want meat every single day of the week and would often threaten to bash up the school cook if he wasn't served more than his frugal ration. And to prove to the cook that he meant business, he'd do a hundred push-ups right there in front of him. Biceps got his meat in a hurry after that. So, I asked my wife to lay out a spread of many chunky meats. I then burnished my best single malts in anticipation of my old friend's arrival and even tried in vain to locate the old album which contained all my school pictures. I couldn't wait.

The big day finally arrived. I had told my office staff that this long lost friend of mine was expected later in the evening, that the red carpet should be laid out for him, and that I should be informed immediately upon his arrival. When they finally announced Biceps, I almost ran out to the waiting area, eager with anticipation, to receive him. I cannot recall when I had last done something like that.

To say that I was shell-shocked would have been the understatement of the millennium. I looked at him and almost recoiled in disbelief. I was staring at a short, pot-bellied, bespectacled old man who I didn't recognise from Adam. I was sure that there was a big mistake somewhere. Was this another patient and not Biceps?

'I do look different than I did in school, don't I Suds?' he said, helpfully. And then, in his old, familiar style, he delivered the backhand jab. 'So do you,' he returned. That settled once for all, any delusions I might have had about my own youthful and well-maintained appearance.

'Yes, I have grown by several inches since you last saw me', I admitted, looking down at him. 'But let's cut the wisecracks. Tell me, what's all this about?'

'Well...man, I've got a file here that's even thicker than my famed biceps of yesteryears. Here, take a look. I've been to every conceivable specialist all over the goddamned world, but they've not been able to solve my problem. Right now, I'm in shit creek: my career, my health, my marriage, you name it; everything's on the rocks. 'Including your scotch whisky,' I thought to myself, priding myself on my brilliant anticipatory diagnosis.

Biceps, now fifty-one, had had a miserable past seven years. A formerly fit and successful business tycoon, things had suddenly started going wrong for him. He had worked hard to achieve everything in life. The hard work must have begun after school, for sure, because I had never seen any signs of it during the time that I knew him! Then, all of a sudden, he lost his father, split with his brothers, his marriage started to fail, his son left home, his business took a major turn for the worse, he got involved in extramarital affairs, started drinking and smoking heavily, stopped exercising, and his health started suffering. He tided over the turbulent phase and stabilised his business and marriage somewhat, but life wasn't ever the same as before. He felt that he was just lying down and watching his life pass him by. He felt chronically fatigued and anxious, couldn't get himself out of bed in the mornings, suffered endless headaches and body aches, sweated excessively, lost his concentration, let umpteen business opportunities slip past him, was constantly irritable, was experiencing problems with his memory, often felt suicidal, and had lost his libido and erection almost completely. None of the medicines that he had taken had helped improve his symptoms. He was currently on high doses of anti-depressants and thought that he had reached the end of the road.

By the time he had finished narrating his tale of woe, he looked miserable and on the verge of tears. I was really feeling very bad for him. He had gone through a bad time. I wanted very much to help him.

I studied his medical reports. The doctors had performed every conceivable test; except one they didn't conceive of – the

Free Androgen Index, or FAI. I wasn't surprised. Even today, most specialists don't understand the entity called andropause (or male menopause), and think that it is just fashionable jargon. This is despite lots of medical evidence to the contrary. Besides, Biceps hadn't really picked the right specialists.

My suspicion turned out to be bang on. Mr Biceps' Free Androgen Index was grossly abnormal. Eight months ago, I started him on testosterone replacement therapy (TRT), and outlined to him many desirable lifestyle changes. Today, he is a drastically transformed man. He is charged, positive, back to work with a renewed enthusiasm, bereft of pains and aches, has resumed exercise, looks fit, and drinks only in moderation, on weekends. His business and marriage are much better too. A truly remarkable comeback, I'd say. Not very common.

Biceps and I are now in fairly regular touch. The last time he called, he told me, 'Hey, you know, my wife thinks I should act in a film,' he said. She says that the film should be called *The Reincarnation of Proud Peter.* 'What do you think? Shall we go for it?' He burst into a long, loud, guffaw.

It must've been ages since he was in such a good mood. I was genuinely happy for him. 'Go for it ma'an,' I played along. 'But don't be too proud of your reincarnated Peter, or he'll peter out again.'

Take Home Message:

It has now been established with certainty that men go through andropause, a mid-life condition quite similar to the menopause in women. Unlike in the woman, however, male sex hormone production does not stop completely in andropause. Instead, there is a tapering. The rate at which this occurs varies from individual to individual. Prevention is always better than cure, and timely pre-emptive steps can facilitate smooth transition without crises. Testosterone replacement therapy becomes necessary in many cases, at least as a short-term measure. The author is a strong proponent of lifestyle modification, yoga, meditation and spirituality for this condition.

Further information on the andropause (also known as the male menopause, viropause, ADAM, PADAM) can be found on *http://www.andropause.in*

9

Self Help is the Best Help

And then there was this young chappie in his early thirties who came to me once. Fidgety and hyperactive he was, with too much surplus energy, I remember quite vividly. 'I have a most unusual complaint, doc,' he began, without preamble. 'In fact, I think it's kind of like the opposite of the stuff you see in your practice. You see, I want to have sex three to four times a day, but my wife doesn't want to have it more than once or twice a week, at most. To say that I am frustrated is the understatement of the century, doc.'

I slowly brought my eyes into focus at a point about two feet behind his head. That's usually what I do when I am concentrating, and thinking hard. It's a vacant, blurry kind of gaze. I was thinking to myself that if this Mr Horny thinks that his is an unusual complaint, then he ain't heard nothing about andrology. Also, I thought, the poor guy is probably clueless that the vast majority of human males are in the same boat as him.

I peered at Mr Horny from over the rim of my spectacles. 'How long has this been an issue?' I wanted to know. Horny thought for a while. 'Actually doc, it all started after the birth of our second child. This was some three years ago. In the early days of our marriage, my wife would be quite enthusiastic about sex. She'd take great trouble to look and talk sexy, would call me at my office and try to seduce me, would get quite bold and naughty at the movies and restaurants, was a tigress in bed, and so on. But now, things are so completely different, it's unbelievable. It's like some very bad joke has been played on me. She looks like an unkempt sexless frump most of the time, and is always making some trivial excuse or the other to avoid sex. I felt quite humiliated when I realised that, on a couple of occasions, I was actually begging her for sex. It's just not fair, doc. I mean, this *volte-face* is just unbelievable. It's almost like she tricked me into having sex with her in the past — just to get herself pregnant. Now, she doesn't give a damn. She might as well have gotten herself some sperms from a sperm bank instead of using me like a sperm donor. The irony is that sperm donors get paid for sperms. Here, it's the other way around. I'm the sucker who's paying for everything. I'm screwed every which way but literally.'

For a moment, my mind went back to my own life, to the time just after our own second child. I shuddered at the memory, and hastily came back to the present. In just those nanoseconds, my forehead was dotted with beads of cold sweat, and Mr Horny was quick to notice it. 'You're sweating, doc,' he observed immediately. 'But it's quite cold here. Are you okay?' I mock-cleared my throat like they do in Hindi movies, and hastily changed the subject. 'Why don't you bring your wife along for a chat?' I suggested, 'I'm sure that she too has a point of view on this.' Mr Horny looked doubtful, but finally agreed. The next day both of them came in to see me.

'Ma'am, do you know what your husband was here to see me about yesterday?'

'Yes doc, he's told me,' she said.

'Well then, what's your take on it?' I wanted to know.

'Ummi...let me begin by honestly conceding that he does have a point, doc. But, you see, he's got sex on his mind all the bl**** time. Any time is sex time for him, whereas I'm not always in the mood for it. It's like he's a chimpanzee or something. He wakes up in the morning, and wants to have sex. He wakes up in the middle of the night, and he wants to have sex. He comes home for lunch, and he wants to have sex. He's just had sex a little while ago, and he wants to have sex again. It's quite frightening actually, that he can't seem to think of anything else. Is it normal to be like this, or is this what they call sex mania? Aren't men in their thirties supposed to be absorbed with their work? Even as 'just' a housewife, I have so much to do. I have two children to look after, servants to supervise, the phone and the doorbell never stop ringing etc. etc., but he just wants to shut the bedroom door all the time and have quickies.'

I thought to myself that she was lucky that Mr Horny at least cared to shut the bedroom door before embarking on his favourite activity. I was trying to imagine the children and the servants trooping into Horny's bedroom during the act. It was an interesting picture. Horny's wife interrupted my reverie rudely.

'It's not like I'm frigid or something, doc. I do enjoy sex, and care about my husband enjoying sex too, but surely there's more to life than just f****** ...oops, I mean sex, all the time. Why can't he realise this? I'm surprised that men like him plan the futures of large corporations. How can he have any time to think of the company when he's so besotted with copulation? Even the company will be screwed, to borrow a phrase from men's lingo.'

I wanted to tell her that her husband was in the elite club of not just corporate presidents, but some American presidents too, but thought that it might be calamitous to do so at this juncture. The lady was enraged enough already. 'Besides, he doesn't do anything to build up desire in me. It wasn't like this before. There was a lot of love and affection in the air, tons of tenderness and romance, and oodles of foreplay too. Nothing like that exists any more. So, nowadays, I'm neither always ready for sex, nor do I always enjoy it. I've had enough of this.'

I then turned to Horny and asked if he had anything to say in his defence about all this. Looking like a goat that's being led to the slaughterhouse, he stared at his fingernails, and scratched the back of his head. I was reminded of Zybyskov in the film, *Amar, Akbar, Anthony*. 'Okay doc, maybe she's not altogether wrong, but what's the solution? Am I supposed to turn celibate or castrate myself at this age?' he was impatient to know, as if all this other discussion was just a waste of time. As far as he was concerned, returning his sex life to its pristine glory was the singular purpose of his visit. This guy certainly had a one-track mind.

Though there are notable exceptions to the contrary, that is, wives not getting as much sex as they want from their partners, mismatched libidos usually follow the Hornies' pattern. It's a testosterone-related thing, and men in the peak of their manhood years will have sex on their minds much of the time. The trick is to admit to the situation, talk about it openly, and work towards mutually acceptable adjustments. One fair method is for both man and wife to come half-way (no, I don't mean 'interrupt your orgasms') — the man should be ready to accept a little less sex, and the woman should be ready for a bit more. Sex needn't always be a hundred per cent 'Come Together' phenomenon. Sometimes, it is all right to pleasure one's partner, even if one isn't in the mood for sex oneself. If there is commitment to monogamy, it is necessary to understand that both partners' needs must be met within the context of marriage itself. This includes the right to *not* have sex. Sex must never be coercive or reluctant. Indelicate handling of the situation at this stage can lead to extramarital affairs or other relationship traumas.

Horny looked at me like all this was easier said than done. This was when I explained to him the age-old formula that many of his predecessors on this planet had used. 'Learn to take matters in your own hands,' I told him, and went on to explain the virtues of masturbatory release. I illustrated how the closed fist is much like a vagina and won't complain if he wants to do it ten or fifteen times. That logic seemed to appeal to him immediately. 'It is a harmless safety valve that'll take your mind off sex for short periods and even help you concentrate on some other work,' I reasoned.

I met Horny and his wife at a party recently. They looked happy together. When asked if they'd sorted out their matter, the wife replied, 'Yes, thanks doc, except that my husband spends a helluva long time in the bathroom nowadays, humming one repetitive old song.'

I turned to Mr Horny with eyebrows raised. He winked mischievously and leaned towards my ear for a conspiratorial whisper. 'I made this song up, doc. It is a corruption of the old original by Salma Agha. It goes something like, *Dil ke armaan moriyon mein beh gaye*' (The desires of the heart have flown down the drains).

I couldn't stop laughing.

Take Home Message:

Libido mismatches among partners are common. It is important to talk about it and to try and work out acceptable solutions. Good communication lines and compromise are of vital importance.

10

Wake up and Smell the Coffee!

One of the fringe benefits of a sub-specialty medical practice is that it gives you a great opportunity to meet different kinds of people: local and foreign, rural and urban, rich and poor, educated and uneducated, young and old. In India, one also gets to meet and study people who speak different languages and practise assorted religions. Thus, every day, one can observe and learn something new. This is also humbling experience, because it makes me realise that there are so many things I don't know.

Let me illustrate this point by telling you about this young man who, long ago, walked into my office, sat down, and began, 'Doc, I have a f***ing problem, a serious f***ing problem!'

I had not had a good day myself. A million annoying things had happened to me since that morning. I wanted to tell him, ' Hey, you think YOU have a f***ing problem, I have a million f***ing problems ma'an, so what's all this bad language for?!'

Instead, I asked him politely, 'Uh, and what might that fffff..., I mean problem, be?'

He seemed like a guy who was not used to wasting his time in order to make himself understood. 'I already told you, doc,' he retaliated brusquely, 'I have a f***ing problem. Aren't you supposed to be the specialist who helps people f***?'

Come to think of it, I had never thought of myself 'that way', but the guy sure had a point. And the fact that he looked so dead serious, only made it that much more difficult for me to keep a straight face.

Not too many people use the word 'f***' so literally. I don't know if you have observed this, but even the most profane of men who use the F word all the time, will usually refer to the act of sexual intercourse euphemistically, especially in a doctor's office. 'Having sex', 'making love', 'makin' out', 'doing it', etc, are a few of these terms. This cool Charlie, however, was certainly different. If anything, it was I who was discomfited.

There's always a first time for everyone, for everything. This was one of those firsts for me. But that was long ago. Since then, I have heard the F word being used by patients many times. It is especially fun when the user is speaking in the vernacular and 'f***' is the only English word in the entire conversation. Like one chap told me, 'Doctor *saab, main jab* f*** *karne jaata hoon na, tab bahut jaldi shot ho jaata hai.* (Sir, when I proceed to f***, I ejaculate very early).' I was new in Hyderabad those days, and, having never heard this term before, was clueless about what this chap was trying to say. I distinctly remember placing a discreet call to a knowledgeable local friend to figure that one out. This friend had spent a considerable part of his life practising the specialty that I merely preach, and explained to me in an instant what this patient was trying to say. 'Shot', apparently, meant ejaculation! Who would have guessed that? Now you know what I meant when I said that specialty medical practice offers many new learning experiences.

If you thought that these were funny, listen to what's next. This time, the user of the 'f***' word was a lady. It is not common for women to use this word in a doctor's office. It's a different matter at home, where women are telling their husbands to 'f*** off!' all the time. That's very common. I'm sure many of you know that very well from first hand experience.

Yes, so we come back to this woman. 'Doc, my husband is very weak in f***ing'. He is out even before he is in,' she told me casually.

This woman was only semi-literate, but was earnest, and was communicating in the best way she knew. She was unaware that 'f***' is considered by most to be a bad word. I couldn't help marvelling that, unbeknown to herself, she had just presented what was perhaps the most succinct case history in andrological history.

Just one word and it can say so much.

Why then, do people make such a big fuss about such a commonly used and expressive word, I thought to myself. Today, many kids use the F word, and many popular songs contain it. In fact, the songs are probably popular mainly because they contain it. I felt that maybe it was time to change our attitude to the word.

When we were children, things were very different. Of course, that was four decades and a lustrum ago, but still, the F word was not unknown. I remember how the really 'bad' boys in class, like me, would go up to the 'good' guys and sing:

> *Father, Uncle, Cousin, King*
> *Went to market on a string*
> *The string broke*
> *What's the joke?!*

Most wouldn't understand a thing, leave alone spot a joke. We'd then have to explain to them that the joke was contained in the first letters of the words on the first line of the song, and that they would have to put these letters together to figure it out. When they finally decoded it, these kids would be completely scandalised and we'd hear a lot of *oohs* and *aahs*, and receive the kind of looks that porn stars would receive at a place of worship.

Things are drastically different today. Recently, at a Sunday lunch party at a friend's place, I heard the host's ten-year-old son Chotu telling his friend, quite loudly, to go 'f***' himself. Many elders were aghast, and the sinning boy's parents reprimanded him quite harshly in front of all the others. The boy started weeping. This infuriated his father even more, and he slapped the boy. The party was ruined.

Incensed by this boorish outburst from the father, Chotu's thirteen-year-old brother sprung to his defence. Pointing to a page in a rather thick book he was holding, he said, 'Dad, please leave him alone! You elders think that you are educated and hip, don't you? Why don't you wake up, smell the coffee, and learn to move with the times? Here, get off your high horse and take a look at this, will you? You might even learn something.'

He was pointing to a page in the *Oxford Advanced Learner's Dictionary*:

The father stared at the page suspiciously at first, but soon got so engrossed that he couldn't let go of the dictionary. After a few minutes, he was rolling with laughter, and had to sit down. Soon, his friends crowded around him and tried to peep over his shoulder into the page all at once. One by one, they all burst

fuch-sia /ˈfjuːʃə/ *n* shrub with red, purple or white drooping flowers.

fuck /fʌk/ *v* (△ *sl*) **1** [I, Tn] have sexual intercourse with (sb). **2** [I, Tn] (esp imperative or as an *interj* in exclamations expressing extreme anger, annoyance or disgust): *Fuck (it)!* ○ *Fuck you — I don't care if I never see you again.* ○ *Fuck the bloody thing — it won't work.* **3** (idm) **'fucking well** (used to emphasize an angry statement, esp an order) certainly; definitely: *You're fucking well coming whether you want to or not.* **4** (phr v) **fuck a'bout/ a'round** behave foolishly or unhelpfully: *Stop fucking around and come and give me a hand.* **fuck sb about/around** treat sb badly or inconsiderately: *This bloody company keeps fucking me about.* **fuck 'off** (esp imperative) go away. **fuck sth up** spoil or ruin sth.

▷ **fuck** *n* (usu *sing*) (△ *sl*) **1** act of sexual intercourse. **2** (*sexist*) person, esp a woman, considered as a sexual partner: *She's a good fuck.* **3** (idm) **not care/give a fuck (about sb/sth)** not care at all: *He doesn't give a fuck about anyone else.*

fucker *n* (△ *sl*) (as a general term of abuse) fool; idiot.

fuck·ing (△ *sl*) *adj, adv* (used to add emphasis in expressions of anger, annoyance, etc): *I'm fucking sick of the whole fucking lot of you.*

▢ **,fuck-'all** *n* [U] (△ *sl*) nothing at all: *You've done fuck-'all today* ○ [attrib] *He's fuck-all ‚use as a 'goalkeeper*

fuck-up /ˈfʌkʌp/ *n* (△ *sl*) complete mess; disaster:

out laughing. After what seemed like an eternity, the formation broke up, and Chotu's father put the dictionary down. His eyes still red and tear-filled after all that laughter, he sent for Chotu.

Chotu was very reluctant to come out at first, but his brother, who was eyewitness to his father's thawing, managed to persuade him. When he finally emerged from his room, it was obvious that Chotu had been crying. 'Come here *beta*,' said the father, 'I'm sorry I f***ed about with your feelings. I admit that it was all a big f*** up.' Will you please forgive me?'

Everybody laughed. The boy knew that his father was eventually always fair. He forgave him readily and they kissed and made up.

'All right guys, let's stop f***ing' around with this party any further. Who's for one more round of Bloody Marys?'

Nobody looked like they wanted to f***'off from there in a hurry after that.

Take Home Message:

The F word may have entered the dictionaries, but, if you look carefully, it is still considered a slang (*sl*) word. So please don't start using it in your office reports or teach your Chotu to use it in his school essay!

11

On Fast Guys and other Seminal Matters

Mankind has forever been obsessed with seminal matters. Miraculous qualities have always been ascribed to this rather ordinary body fluid by nearly every culture in human history. Almost everyone has heard sometime or the other the fantastic 'fact' that one drop of semen equals forty drops of blood. (This is only a conservative average guesstimate!) Hence, it is rather surprising that the human race hasn't bled itself into extinction by now, given the enormous volumes of seminal fluid that are lost every day in every part of the world.

The total quantity of a man's semen has been assumed to be a valuable lifetime constant from which all release has to be rationed very frugally. It is almost like every man comes down from the heavens with just one *lota* (small urn) of semen, his pre-determined quota. Though this hypothetical 'constant' quantity has never really been determined, and the quotas for rationed release never specified, loss of semen has nonetheless been associated with debility. Even today, it is not uncommon to see educated, successful, widely travelled men complaining of severe 'total body weakness' and assorted debilities from head to toe because they believe that they have lost too much semen. Quacks and fraudulent sexologists help quite considerably in perpetrating this myth. In fact, for many, this myth is very necessary for their livelihood.

The roots of this phenomenon can probably be traced to a heinous conspiracy that has been hatched by family elders and clergymen aeons ago. What must have actually begun as a petty scare to keep sexually errant males in tow, eventually became a widespread and deeply entrenched belief across most cultures. This explains why many members of the medical profession are not exempt from this belief either. When a doctor himself/herself believes that loss of semen causes 'weakness', what chance does the poor patient have?

It is interesting to note that women, who actually lose measurable quantities of menstrual blood every month, do not suffer from any such weaknesses.

'But is there no truth whatsoever in these beliefs about semen?' I can still hear the sceptics among you ask, incredulously. The answer is an emphatic 'No!' Seminal fluid is a dynamic body fluid. It is produced by the body with one express purpose, *viz.* expulsion from the body to the exterior. Semen cannot be conserved and stored inside the body for indefinitely long periods, no matter how hard a man might try. The glands **that** store semen are very small and have a capacity of only a few millilitres. They have to be emptied regularly so that freshly produced semen might take the place of effete semen. If the semen is not expelled into the vagina by intercourse, and not even released by masturbation, it will automatically find its way out as nocturnal emissions during sleep anyway. There is no way that seminal fluid can be kept locked up inside the body. Semen is not produced from blood either, like many have been erroneously led to believe. Furthermore, the vital component in semen, the spermatozoa or sperms, have a finite life span, and, if not utilised for fertilisation of the ovum in that time, will perish. Semen is thus, just a fluid produced by the body for release to the outside, like sweat, urine and tears. It is intended by nature to be routinely thrown out of the body, without any deleterious consequences whatsoever. Yet, myths about semen loss induced debility abound to an extent that seriously affects the well-being of human males all over the world. I see men every day, from all cultures and strata, presenting some kind of complaint related to loss of semen. Some come in trembling, some come with severe anxiety–depression, some, who are students, have failed the same exam several times, some are unable to marry until this 'weakness' is cured, some have become 'impotent' because of excessive masturbation, some feel electric shocks going down their spine because they've lost too much semen, some have lost twenty kilograms of weight, some have become totally anorectic, some have developed severe 'nervous weakness' — you name the symptom, and I'll show you evidence that somewhere, someone is blaming masturbation for having caused it. It is hardly surprising, therefore, that quacks are having a rollicking time, and are laughing their way to the banks.

Another semen-related condition that is very poorly understood by most laymen is ejaculation. Though ejaculation often occurs normally, and is an intensely pleasurable and straight-forward experience for most men, it is actually an extremely complex phenomenon that is regulated by many different systems.

Erotic films and literature depicting 'bucketfuls of cum' squirted several feet by monstrous phalluses can flummox even the best-informed. The magnitude of sexual misinformation that's floating around is unbelievable. One educated guy actually told me, 'C'mon doc, are you trying to tell me that all of it is trick videography? How can anyone fake penis size, for God's sake? They're showing the whole man in the shots, not just his penis. And they actually show the semen gushing out from the tip of the penis. In fact, the camera zooms in on it. How can you say that all of it is make-believe, doc? You're just saying it to make me feel good.'

What could I say...? Some misconceptions are so deep-rooted.

Let's take a look at premature ejaculation (PE), also known as early orgasmic response. PE is extremely common. Kinsey, in his landmark report, had stated that it affects seventy-five per cent of all men. Premature ejaculation is especially relevant today because of the increasing hype about female sexual gratification. The new-millennium woman, it seems, will not take anything lying down unless it is long-lasting enough.

However, PE seems to be nature's original design. The *Kama Sutra* has, in fact, classified PE as one of several normal ejaculatory patterns. PE actually seems to confer an evolutionary procreative advantage on humans. Early man's environs were dangerous and he often had very little time in which to impregnate his partner and ensure propagation of the species. The continuation of this atavistic PE streak perhaps explains the preponderance of the condition in modern man. It appears, in fact, that the ability to prolong ejaculation time has to be learnt, and that it does not come naturally to humans. Masters and Johnson described exercises for this thirty years ago. Today, in many societies in many parts of the world, there is more recreative sex than procreative sex on the whole, and men do not have Darwinian excuses for their premature ejaculation any longer.

The spectrum of PE is vast. Some men ejaculate at the mere thought of coitus. For such people, sex is truly just 'between the ears'. Others last long enough by average standards but are yet unable to gratify their partners. There are many reasons for this. Female sexual gratification is quite complex and is more than just a function of peno-vaginal thrusting and ejaculatory competence. Therefore, men must acquire additional love-making skills.

Attempts have been made to measure PE objectively using many different methods. Researchers have actually placed stop-watches and pelvic thrust counters in patients' bedrooms! None of these methods, however, has proved ideal. The American Psychiatric Association's DSM IV defines PE as 'persistent or recurrent ejaculation with minimal stimulation before, during, or after penetration and before the patient wishes it'. Even this hasn't been standardised. Many additional parameters, notably the importance of physical factors (increasingly incriminated in PE) need to be incorporated. It is now known that injury to the sympathetic nervous system (for example, following surgery for abdominal aortic aneurysm), pelvic fractures, prostatic hypertrophy and prostatitis, urethritis, diabetes, arteriosclerosis, cardiovascular disease, local genito-urinary disease, sensory impairment, polycythemia and polyneuritis can all cause PE.

Despite claims to the contrary, PE can be extremely difficult to treat. Every system of medicine, and every culture boasts its own unique 'cures' for the condition. Since PE is often a psychological disorder, even substances without any real pharmacological effect on the ejaculatory apparatus can seem to work by the mere power of suggestion (placebo). Some decades ago, psychosexual treatment methods gained tremendous popularity. One such was the 'start–stop' method, which was popularised by Semans and Helen Singer Kaplan. The other was the 'squeeze' technique described by Masters & Johnson. These held sway for many decades, largely because of the unavailability of other treatment methods. However, the initial success rates claimed with these were not sustainable and, over a period of time, the success rates had dwindled to twenty-five per cent. Besides, these techniques are very tedious to employ and unsuitable for today's supersonic age.

Nowadays, research is centred on understanding the central and peripheral neurological control of the ejaculatory process and regulating it with drugs. The various treatment options available for PE today include correction of underlying causes, pharmacological therapy (some new promising drugs are coming up), topical applications, psychological treatment and, more recently, even microsurgery.

Pleasure, alas, truly doesn't seem available in an instant.

Take Home Message:

Myths about the deleterious consequences of semen loss abound. All of these are baseless. Loss of semen does NOT cause any weakness.

Premature ejaculation (PE) is the commonest sexual dysfunction. Causes can be both psychological and physical. Many treatment options are available, including new effective oral drugs.

For information on ejaculatory disorders, check out *http://www.anejaculation.com*

12

Not Sohail, I'm Sohaila

Some years ago, a burkha-clad lady from a neighbouring country came to see me. She was accompanied by her identically attired mother. When she lifted her veil to speak, I couldn't help noticing that she was absolutely gorgeous and that she used make-up very skilfully indeed.

'I'm Sohaila, doctor,' she* began, with flawless diction, 'though my given name is Sohail. I am a male-to-female transsexual and have come to you for a sex change operation. These are not being performed in my country.' As she spoke, it became clear to me that this lady was like a walking–talking

---

*It is customary to use the psycho–emotional gender term (rather than the physical gender term) while referring to transsexuals. Thus, a physically male but psycho–emotionally female transsexual will be referred to as 'she' and 'her', and vice versa. The abbreviations MTF and FTM are used to refer to Male to Female transsexuals and Female to Male transsexuals, respectively.

encyclopaedia on the subject of transsexualism and gender reassignment surgery. It is amazing what some education and access to the internet can do, I thought to myself.

Just a few years ago, Sohaila was on the verge of committing suicide. She had faced humiliation and ostracism all her life and was always thought to be a freak. The kindest judgement of her was that she was a pansy, or a homosexual. Even some of the doctors who saw her could not understand that this was a woman who was trapped in a man's body. She was despised and thought to be a curse by her father and brothers. The one person who stood by her like the proverbial rock through all this, however, was her mother, whose support was unconditional and unstinting. With her encouragement, Sohaila dropped out of school, pursued her education privately, and fared brilliantly. Subsequently, she completed her Bachelor's, and Master's as well. And that's when she started researching her own condition on the internet.

'When I first started surfing the internet, doctor,' she said, 'I used to break down and cry quite frequently. The kind of scientific advances and support systems in some of the developed nations are so awesome. Even governments and insurance schemes support transsexuals in some places. Sure, these countries still have some way to go too, but in my part of the world, even this much is unthinkable. I had to hide behind the four walls of my house like a leper, too ashamed to go out. Doctors in my country wouldn't even want to see me for serious medical ailments. Luckily, my parents had some doctor friends, or I don't know what would have happened to me when I suffered all those illnesses as a child. Anyway, through the internet I finally learnt that sex can be changed by operation. I have also seen some 'after operation' pictures on some sites and have read stories of successfully rehabilitated patients who have settled down in meaningful relationships. I too want to be like them, doctor. I have suffered enough.'

She choked on her words and began to cry. Neither her mother nor I interrupted her. The mother merely placed a reassuring palm on Sohaila's back. Both she and I instinctively understood that these were tears of relief. Sohaila needed to get the pain out of her system. We empathised completely and knew what toll all her trials and tribulations must've taken on her. It was not an easy journey for this man–woman; fighting oppression, obtaining information, and finally seeking a solution. Finally, a psychologist in a big town in her country had referred my name to her. She traced me through the internet and wrote to me for an appointment. Truly awesome. It has never ceased to amaze me, to what extent motivated transsexuals will go to in order to find a solution to their condition.

When she finally calmed down, I proceeded to the business of explaining her case to her. 'Before I start, Sohaila,' I began, 'I must warn you that you have not by any means reached the end of your journey. In fact, you have taken just one major first step. There's still a long way to go. Are you prepared? Operation and conversion of the genitalia from masculine to feminine is just one stage, albeit a very important one, of the treatment programme. There are many other important components too. Many patients get disillusioned because they are not told of all the hardships involved, right at the outset. They are just shown pictures of outstandingly beautiful women after operation and are told that they can become like that. The many steps along the way are conveniently omitted. This is not how I'd like to do it. I'd like to tell you everything, not so that I dissuade you from going through it, which is not in my interest either, but so that you may make a well-informed choice, and be strong. Are you ready, Sohaila?'

'I see your point, doctor. No unrealistic expectations from me. I am a realist. Tell me the facts as they are.'

I spoke to Sohaila at length. I explained to her that the first step is a thorough psychosexual evaluation, then hormone therapy, and that surgery starts after that. I told her that total transformation will involve multiple steps, and that she has already taken the first step by dressing and living like a lady.

'Many MTF transsexuals come here in trousers, with thick beards, gruff voices, and prominent Adam's apples and expect us to work miracles. How can we?! You are lucky in that sense. From what little I can see of your face, neck and hands, you seem to be quite non-hairy. That's definitely an advantage,' I explained.

Hormone therapy, which has to be stopped three months before operation, I told her, was the first step. Hormones are necessary to start the feminisation process. Later, when the testes are removed as part of the surgery, the male hormone testosterone gets cut off, and the feminisation progresses faster. Often, body hair gets sparse and scanty with this much alone, and breast development, too, is adequate in some. Many others will require, or desire, breast implants. For the hair, in some cases, prolonged sessions of laser therapy and/or electrolysis become necessary. Even after that, some hair removal may be required on a regular basis. The use of makeup needs to be mastered too. I told Sohaila that I could see that this is another area where she has made great progress. She blushed and dropped her gaze coyly.

'And then', I told her, 'there's the issue of the Adam's apple. Sometimes, surgery is required to surgically reduce its prominence. Again, that's not very pertinent to your case though. Lastly, there's the matter of the voice. On occasion, vocal cord surgery is performed to make it more feminine, but this becomes optional or even unnecessary if the voice is sufficiently feminine. Of course, one can go on and on endlessly. Nose jobs, total chest recontouring, buttocks' padding...you name it, it can be done. But the expenditure, duration of hospitalisation, emotional toll, etc., all add up. Few go all the way, though. Many are in stable relationships already by the time they come to us, and have partners who already accept them unconditionally even before sex change surgery, so that makes it a lot easier and better for all concerned. Do you have a partner already, Sohaila?'

'No doctor, I'm not ready for a partner yet. You see, I'm not a transvestite or a homosexual. So, until and unless my genitalia are changed, taking a partner is unthinkable to me. It's not as if I haven't had my fair share of admirers though, despite my exposure to the outside world being so limited. But they'll all have to wait.'

I admired her clarity of thought. The rest of the consultation progressed rapidly. It's not frequently that one sees such psycho-emotionally balanced MTF transsexuals. Often, their psychological state itself requires working on quite a bit before surgery. By comparison, Sohaila was exceptionally balanced. She was also very feminine in her musculoskeletal appearance, body hair, and voice aspects; every gender reassignment surgeon's dream. I posted her for early surgery.

We performed the genital and breast operations on Sohaila on the same day at the same sitting. Both went off well and she was discharged in ten days after a smooth recovery. Much of this was also thanks to her stoical disposition towards pain and discomfort. Trauma since childhood, and time, had inured her.

She stayed in touch with me every month after that, and sometimes even in between, for this and that. Each month, she would email me pictures of the operated areas and the scar areas. They were all progressing well.

When she finally came back for a checkup after six months (she had taken hormones meantime), I couldn't even recognise her. She walked in wearing jeans and a *kurta*, and her appearance had changed quite considerably. Sohaila had also filled out a bit with a female type fat distribution, and looked a lot more feminine. Only a very trained eye could have told that she was a gender reassigned MTF transsexual. I was very happy for her.

'Can I start having sex, doctor?' she asked, with a matter of fact forthrightness. After I examined her and gave her the green signal, she told me that she was already seeing someone, and was planning to get married. 'He loves me a lot, doctor,' she said, 'He doesn't care that I can never have children. We have decided that we will adopt children. I don't know how to thank you.'

I should be thanking you, I thought to myself. We can't produce such great results every time in sex change surgery. Sohaila's case was exceptional — every gender reassignment surgeon's dream case. I was happy for both of us.

She walked away, and never looked back in life again after that.

For further information on transsexualism, the reader is referred to *http://www.transsexualism.co.in*

13

Re-opening Closed Chapters

This case history is now quite a few years old. A young couple had come to consult me. The man and the wife were both young, in their early thirties. They were well dressed, articulate and seemed highly educated. Yet, something about them was curiously unusual. There was a distinct aura of gloom and melancholia surrounding them.

This, in itself, is not uncommon in my practice. The gloom, I mean. Couples struggling with infertility and erectile dysfunction are often depressed, and their relationships too, are precariously balanced, if not altogether jeopardised. But this couple's sadness seemed to belong in a different category. They seemed so fragile that it was hard for me to decide whether I should break the ice or wait for them to speak. I was afraid that I might say the wrong thing and trigger off something inadvertently. My empathy was instantaneous.

The couple's inter-personal relationship didn't seem one bit estranged though. The looks they exchanged were that of deep love and understanding. It was almost as if they were together in their grief, with an even stronger bonding than in fun times. There was definitely some other issue at play here, an issue on which I was not able to put my finger immediately. Sensitivity and delicacy were the need of the hour, my antennae warned me.

'Yes, please,' I finally began because they didn't, 'what can I do for you?'

'Ours is a somewhat unfortunate case, doctor,' the husband replied. 'My wife and I are both highly qualified working professionals. We got married about six years ago. Ours was a dream marriage of sorts, with everything falling into place, like a fairy tale. We met at the workplace, fell in love, and after a few months' brief whirlwind courtship, got married with our parents' whole-hearted approval. Both our families are affluent and there was nothing missing in our lives. Within a year and a half of our marriage, we were blessed with a bonny son. Our joy knew no bounds. Then, when our son was two years old, we decided that with both of us being so career-minded, we didn't want another child. My wife and I discussed it pretty much in detail, and I underwent a vasectomy.'

He paused. By now, his wife was choking on stifled sobs. Just the trigger I was afraid I might accidentally pull, I thought to myself. To her credit, however, she recovered quickly and regained her composure.

I knew what was coming next. I have been through case histories like this a couple of times in the past. However, the correct thing for me to do was to wait until they told me. If I was wrong, it would have been even more calamitous, so I waited for them to tell me. I could feel their pain as they relived their traumatic experience all over again, but could do nothing but wait and let them take their time to finish. After a brief while, they regained their composure somewhat.

'Six months ago,' the husband continued, 'we lost our only child in a tragic accident. We didn't imagine in our wildest dreams that such a tragedy could befall us when I went in for a vasectomy. How we take simple things for granted! Nothing is in our hands, actually. Our lives have turned completely upside down after that, doctor. Nothing, nothing in life hereafter can ever compensate us for this irreparable loss.'

I waited for them to settle down after the hardest part. I took a deep breath too. I admired their fortitude. Such a young couple, and all this just when their lives seemed picture perfect. It didn't take long for them to recover. This time, the wife spoke, finally.

'We are slowly coming to terms with what has happened to us, doctor, but the void in our lives is simply too much to bear. We are now very keen to have another child. I have spoken to my gynaecologist about this, and she has suggested an In Vitro Fertilisation (IVF)/Intra Cytoplasmic Sperm Injection (ICSI) procedure as the best solution to our predicament. She said that they would retrieve sperms from my husband's testes using a needle or a biopsy procedure, and then inject the sperm directly into my egg at the time of ovulation. But my husband, who has surfed the internet extensively on the subject and has also read many of your columns in the past, seems to be convinced that we have a better chance of success with a microsurgical vasectomy reversal operation. That's why we are here, doc. We don't know what to do.'

'You are placing an unfair responsibility on me,' I told them. 'I can only explain to you the various available options, and tell you what the success rates, costs, hospital stay duration, and other logistics are. The final decision will have to be made by you.'

'We're okay with that doctor. I know you will tell us the facts right.'

Most doctors would have been flattered with such trust from a patient. I always get a bit apprehensive instead. I am notorious for warning patients about all the gory morbid details of every procedure. I don't tell them that a particular procedure carries a seventy-five per cent success rate. I tell them instead that it carries a twenty-five per cent failure rate. When they ask if it'll hurt, I say, 'Yes! It certainly will.' In the beginning of my practice, I was warned, and therefore worried, that I might lose patients because I am so blunt. However, to my pleasant surprise, I found that my patients not only appreciated my honesty and thanked me for it, they also coped with their post-operative situation much better. For instance, most patients experience less pain than they had been told to expect, and this improves their convalescence quite considerably. Therefore, to cut a long story short, this couple couldn't have been more right when they said that I would tell them the facts right!

I pointed them to many articles from leading international textbooks and journals, including one from the then current issue of the revered journal, *Fertility & Sterility*, which clearly mentioned that the results of a microsurgically performed vasectomy reversal operation are superior to those obtained with IVF techniques if the reversal is performed at centres of excellence. The results are even better if the vasectomy reversal is performed within five years of the vasectomy. The patency rates can exceed ninety per cent and the pregnancy rates, seventy per cent. Besides, the whole exercise is cheaper than one cycle of IVF and is a one-time day care surgery. The patient spends only a few hours in the hospital.

On the other hand, I pointed out, even the cumulative success rates of IVF/ICSI after several cycles cannot match these figures at most centres. Besides, each cycle entails visits for the woman to the IVF centre for several days, many medicines and injections, serial ultrasound scans, and an ovum pick up. At the end of all this, the success rates are only a modest fifteen to twenty per cent per cycle even at the best centres. The procedure will have to be performed three to six times if the success rates have to equal that obtained with a microsurgical vasectomy reversal operation. And there is a high cost involved each time too.

Another great thing about a microsurgical vasectomy reversal, I told them, is that when it works, enduring results can be expected, and one can even have many children in the future. By contrast, IVF/ICSI procedures have to be repeated each time, and each attempt costs more than a microsurgical vasectomy reversal operation.

'Thanks for the reassurance, doc. This is exactly what I showed my wife on the internet. I took her to the sites of the best infertility microsurgery centres in the world, but her doctor didn't agree with those figures.'

'There may be a reason for that,' I told them. 'Not all infertility surgeons are trained to perform microsurgery. Many will just use optical loupes (magnifying spectacles) and loosely call it microsurgery. The two are totally different, and so are the results. Your doctor must be speaking from experience with such surgery and its poor results. But all reversal operations are not alike; microsurgery is different. It employs magnifications of up to forty times and allows for great precision. By contrast, most loupes offer only modest magnifications of three to four times. This is definitely not good enough for the very minute vas deferens, and this is promptly reflected in the poor results. That is probably what your doctor is talking about.'

After two days, the couple came back to me and announced that they have decided to opt for the microsurgical operation. The patient was admitted in the morning, operated upon, and discharged the same evening. Six months after operation, the patient's sperm counts were respectable. They improved steadily, and after a year and a half, the wife conceived again.

They plan to name the baby Amar.

Take Home Message:

Vasectomy can be reversed. When performed microsurgically at centres of excellence, the results are excellent. It is a day care operation, which is performed under local or regional anaesthesia. The results of this reversal operation are usually much superior to the results of IVF/ICSI, if performed at centres of excellence. For these reasons, vasectomy is the sterilisation operation of choice.

14

Are My Macho Days Over?!

Many middle-aged men come to see me, troubled that their macho days are over. Few are cognisant of, or prepared for, the normal changes in male sexuality that accompany ageing. A large fraction of these men also erroneously believes that age is just a 'state of mind', that chronology has nothing to do with it, and that a man's sexuality remains unchanged even in the seventies and eighties. They thus attribute their present depleted sexual state to stress, or a stale relationship, or a passing phase, without even trying to understand the medical facts. Braggadocio claims made by some impotent oldies who boast that they can have sex every day, only obscure the picture further for others. Several men, even the educated ones, have fallen prey to useless medication in the quack or aphrodisiac market for these reasons. After many years, when nothing has worked, they come to me. Otherwise, the usual joke at parties is, 'Doc, you are one specialist I hope I never have to come to.' The irony is that, despite such resolve, many eventually do. They land up at my office when they have finally come to terms with reality, have realised that this phase just doesn't pass, and are convinced that aphrodisiacs are not working for them! By this time usually, a lot of water has already flown under the bridge.

So, what are the sexual problems of middle and old age? What can be considered a normal, age-related change, and what is abnormal?

Let's talk about normal changes first.

The first of these is that elderly men do not get aroused instantaneously, as they did in their younger years. One Mr Sexually Sluggish, aged fifty-eight, told me, 'Doc, I am finished. The kind of chicks that gave me instant hard-ons when I was younger, don't do anything to me now. I'm sure I am becoming impotent. Earlier, if a beautiful babe merely walked past, I'd get horny as a beast. Just the sight, the thought, or the scent of a woman would unleash the lust in me. Touch, of course, was something else. Why that, I'd get erections even on bus rides and in autos just like that, like some vibrator was applied to my dick or something, without anything sexual happening in my mind even. I would need periodic sexual release even in college and in the office because I could not concentrate on my studies or work for too long because of uncontrollable satyriasis. I would have to sneak a stealthy visit to the loo every now and then to perform the needful. Oh, those were the days! They are history now, of course. Extinct. Just like the bloody dinosaurs. Nothing arouses me instantly any more. My poor partner has to work hard on my limp penis to awaken it. Often, it takes so much time that both of us lose interest, and don't want to continue the traumatic charade any longer. I feel terrible for her, doc. I am still very skilled with my fingers and tongue, but can they substitute for the real thing ? We both know that it is a pathetic situation. Give me something to pep me up, doc. It's going from bad to worse. And you know one more thing, doc? My wife's considerably younger than I am, and still very attractive, and is out at work all day. Sometimes, I get so insecure that she'll stray, I feel a wrenching pain in my gut. I'm only human doc, and she too.' He sounded really miserable.

'Tell me,' I finally had a chance to jump in, 'When you do get aroused finally, how are the erection, the performance, and the satisfaction quotient of both partners?'

'Disastrous doc, I just told you. Weak initial rigidity, no sustenance, no ejaculation, no partner orgasm. Everything is a disaster.'

I reassured him and proceeded to explain that sexuality changes with age, and that what he was going through was not unusual, and that millions of men the world over go through the same things. 'After a particular age, men finally learn to think with the right heads,' I tried to light-heartedly reassure him. I was not telling him the whole truth, of course. It is certainly not normal for all elderly men to be totally impotent, but I didn't want to break the bad news to him yet.

Many men are not easily reconciled though. Some men think that a younger woman might be able to recapture the magic for them. They get embroiled in affairs with younger women, womanise serially, or marry kids young enough to be their daughters. No matter what the chosen escape option is, there is usually a considerable toll on the man's financial resources. The expenses incurred are usually directly proportional to the size of the bedroom debacles. Some other men try pornography or splurge money on aphrodisiacs. Needless to say, all this still doesn't solve their problem, and they come back for medical help.

I went on to tell Mr Sluggish about the other changes accompanying ageing. One of these, I told him, is the ejaculatory experience. With age, both the intensity and the volume of ejaculation can reduce. This again, is a source of major perturbation for many men. Thus, a man who could proudly squirt his semen a few feet ahead in his heydays, gets a rude shock when the squirt gets reduced to a mere ooze, a drop, or sometimes nothing at all. Besides, the whole ejaculatory experience itself becomes much less intense, and is no longer 'mind-blowing' or 'earth-shattering' like it used to be. In fact, quite often, the middle-aged man is content not ejaculating at all, and actually abandons coitus without doing so even though his erection is good. That overpowering urge to release pent up sexual tension and semen is simply no longer there. This actually perplexes both him, and his partner, but is again just a variation of the normal. Some years ago, such a sexual response would have been unthinkable to the same man. The vascular congestion of the sexual organs consequent upon sexual arousal in both the sexes is so severe in younger ages, that not attaining climax can actually cause congestive pains in the genital regions and other symptoms elsewhere. Many young men who lack sexual opportunity and who believe that masturbation is harmful and causes weakness, chronically suffer from such pains. Sexual release is the only cure for this.

However, all this changes considerably as the man ages.

Another sexual area of concern to the middle-aged man is the refractory period, or the interval between erections. At eighteen or twenty, a man is ready for sex a second time within minutes. With age, this changes a lot too, and some men cannot get another erection for much longer periods. Some men will not get another erection for several days after one ejaculation. A few elderly men are able to make their first and only erection last much longer. Many also report delayed rather than premature ejaculation. Thus, some sprinters of yore become marathon men, but remain athletes nonetheless. However, not all elderly men can do this. In fact, more than half of all men over the age of forty will have some degree of erectile dysfunction (impotence).

With age, the angle of the erection also changes. In young boys and young men, erections are nearly vertical and almost touch their lower abdominal walls. With age, the 'angle of the dangle' reduces, and you can be said to be doing well if the erection is at or just above the horizontal. Of course, it goes without saying that you are in deep trouble and need urgent help if your aroused apparatus points to the ground. If it's limp as well, then that would constitute a really major dual fiasco.

There are other hormone-related changes in the ageing male too. These affect various organ systems in the body and are clubbed together under the term 'andropause' or 'male menopause'. This is discussed in another chapter.

It is important that more men understand these bodily changes and come to terms with a sexuality that is age appropriate. Too many men are either needlessly languishing in misery or trying to compensate for their waning manhood by posing as macho studs in their middle age. Remember, even top level athletes and sportsmen in many fields retire when they are only in their twenties and thirties. Physical fitness always fades after a particular age. It is inevitable.

You must be wondering what happened to Mr Sexually Sluggish. Well, I conducted some tests on him. These revealed that he did not have any major medical condition like diabetes, high blood pressure, high cholesterol or very low testosterone, but he did have considerably reduced blood flow to his penis. I tried the new wonder drugs on him but they worked only partially. I finally suggested surgery, which gives excellent results, but, like many Indian men, he is petrified of the scalpel and is taking his own time to make up his mind. Meantime, he is using a vacuum device (an external device used to induce erection), with the help of which he seems to be doing at least something.

I hope that many of you are feeling much better now, after reading all this. You may now put away your protractors!

Take Home Message:

Male sexuality goes through different phases as a man ages. Unfortunately, on account of various prevailing myths and misinformation, these phases are very poorly understood. A correct understanding of what constitutes age-appropriate sexuality, and what constitutes an andrological disease state is important so that one may take timely action if necessary. Since both disease states and physiological changes can co-exist in middle age and beyond, it is important to recognise the difference. Physiological changes are to be lived with, whereas pathological states will require treatment.

15

Basic Instinct? Or Learned Behaviour?

People sometimes ask me which is more important to human sexuality: basic instinct, or learned behaviour. Some argue that sex in humans is primal, instinctive behaviour and doesn't require any teaching. Such people believe that sex education is not only unnecessary but also buncombe. They argue that the whole concept of sex education is recent and that humans have been copulating and reproducing for millennia without the need for such garbage. Besides, they state, nobody teaches animals how to make love. Yet, they point out, you can see animals of all kinds copulating freely if you walk through the streets of a city (in India, of course!) or the countryside, and that's how natural and spontaneous sex was meant to be.

On the other hand, at the other end of the spectrum there are people who have gone through experiences where, for example, their son-in-law hadn't consummated his marriage with their daughter in several months because he did not even know how and where to put it in! There are several other such situations where the sexual debacles are directly related to sexual ignorance. I see these in my practice every day. People who are involved in these situations will be ready to swear that if only there had been proper sex education, all this would never have happened.

So, which is it? Instinct? Or education?

Good question.

Actually, now that Mr Cave Man is extinct, it is more of the latter and less of the former, if you ask me. The sexual instinct in humans is unarguably primal, animalistic, and, except perhaps where there is disease or dysfunction, very strong. However, while such an instinct is crucial for the propagation of the species, it carries with it many other attendant ramifications and complications.

And that's both the problem and challenge for mankind.

Unlike in the animal kingdom, sexual behaviour in civilised humans is controlled by man-made laws. To add to this are moral, cultural, and religious mores. Even these are not homogenous and vary across cultures and religions, thus making matters that much more complex in a seamless, global environment.

In many ways, man-made laws are not only good, but also necessary or one would find humans blissfully copulating randomly and acrobatically on the streets and countryside all the time. There would be no husbands, no wives. Nobody would know who their father is. Men would gouge out each other's innards to win women. And just one person with a sexually transmitted disease (STD) would be enough to infect an entire commune. And so on.

However, it is equally true that too much organised sexuality goes against basic biology. The result is that most humans are unsure about what is normal, healthy, acceptable, and right, and are in constant conflict with their urges. Those that dare to transgress conventional barriers often end up regretting the consequences. In India, for instance, we are exposed to sexual and moral hypocrisies in our indigenous movies on the one hand and, at the same time, have access to western soaps and cinema wherein anything and everything is happening. Not only do we hear about scandals in our immediate environment, we also watch the world exonerating an American president and other celebs for their 'sexcapades'.

What will our children learn?!

All this is genuinely confusing, and makes a strong case for formal sex education (learned behaviour) at the grassroots level at an appropriate age. Sex education is not merely the imparting of trite (and boring) information about menstruation, and showing children two-dimensional reproductive anatomy and physiology diagrams of 'how babies are born'. It should go much deeper than that. The undeniably quintessential nature of sex in human life should be placed in proper perspective. Hype should be differentiated from reality. It should be hammered home that though sex is important, it is not all-important.

Human beings will not die without sex. Sex is not like food or water. It is possible to live without sex. It is certainly not necessary to embrace unsafe or dysfunctional sex at any cost in order to survive. If sexual deprivation can cause emotional and mental problems, we must recognise that dysfunctional sex can cause much greater damage.

People should be taught to use sex in a healthy and responsible manner to fulfil their (and their partners') physical, emotional and reproductive needs. They should be made familiar with societal and marital laws. They should be informed about both conventional and unconventional sexuality and make informed choices about what they wish to embrace. The risks and consequences of aberrant behaviour must also be made known. Partners' needs and duties should be discussed. Spouses should be taught to espouse a moral code that is mutually acceptable to both partners.

And much more...

Ideally, all these should be understood by people before their first sexual experience in order for sex to become more than just a 'basic instinct' curiosity and transform itself into man's most advanced benchmark of evolution, civilisation and culture.

This brings us finally to the sexual act itself, not because it is least important, but because physical sex should be engaged in only after all other aspects have been clearly understood. Otherwise, what's the difference between the naked masturbating chimpanzees in the zoo and us? Good love-making skills are undoubtedly important to a mutually satisfying sex life and should be learnt. These can be picked up from several scientific treatises on the subject, though readers must be cautioned that many of these manuals depict sex in a very clinical manner and all eroticism has to be imagined by the reader. For this reason, unfortunately, no one really reads a sex manual until one's sex life is in a crisis and the book is prescribed as a form of treatment. This only increases the sexlessness of the manual. It also probably explains why most people prefer to acquire their sex skills from Harold Robbins, porn material, and self-proclaimed sex gurus in their coterie instead.

However, the last brand of 'sex education' can be misleading because all women don't attain multiple orgasms in race cars travelling at 100 mph, and all men don't go on all night like relentless battering rams with twelve-inch long penises like in every porn film you've seen. Sorry to disappoint you folks, but real life sex is a lot different than reel life sex.

Sex is also a serious responsibility. Transcending basic instinct is the challenge. And it's time that human beings took that up seriously. Humans have many instincts and urges. Hunger, for instance, is one, but yet, hunger does not have to mean gluttony. Similarly, thirst does not have to mean dipsomania. Likewise, sexual urges don't have to mean satyriasis, rape, other sex crimes and perversions. Many misinformed youngsters today are engaged in the pursuit of precisely such dangerous highs.

Therefore, I believe that just like in other walks of life, sexual behaviour must also be governed by self-restraint and man made laws. After all, civilisation is all about orderly behaviour, within the ambit of laws and practices, which defines the difference between humans and animals. Sex ought not to be an exception. Stating that the basic instinct component of sex is more important than its learned behaviour component is like making a case for animalism in human sexuality.

This probably explains why sexual misbehaviour and crimes in humans are often forgiven but crimes emanating from poverty and a survival instinct are not.

This is morally wrong and reprehensible.

16

Penis Transplants

In clinical practice, doctors often encounter a distinct sub-population of patients who think they know it all. These patients have such strong pre-conceived notions about their illness that you really wonder why they have come to you and why they have not treated themselves and got cured. These patients don't come to ask you about their problem. They come instead to tell, even teach you, about it. In the interesting field of andrology, one often hears patients proffering convoluted and irrational explanations for their sexual condition. Like one guy was telling me how masturbating with the right hand has caused his penis to bend to the right. Another chap explained how lying on his tummy and rubbing his penis on the mattress has caused the penis to become thin and weak. Yet another fellow tried to convince me that his nocturnal emissions (loss of semen by ejaculation during sleep) have caused him to fail in all his exams for five consecutive years!

There's no point telling these men anything to the contrary. We doctors are supposed to simply accept their theories of causation and their self-made diagnoses, and merely do what we are told, *viz.* fix the problem! That's all they want. They don't want us pontificating about the etiopathogenesis (etiology+pathogenesis) of their condition, about which they think we know buzz all nothing. To some of these people, I am, after all, just an allopathic physician. What would I know about the centuries' old wisdom of traditional systems of medicine?

I know only too well how to handle these types. Over the years, I've learnt, and evolved my own methodology. So, here's how one consultation went one afternoon:

'Doctor Krishnamurti,' this guy began, 'my dick has become damn small. I think it is all those years of masturbation and womanising.'

'How do you know how small is small?' I asked him, deliberately ignoring his theories of causation for reasons outlined above.

'I'm telling you, doc. I just know,' he replied.

'Has anybody told you this? How many penises have you seen?' I countered.

That took him a bit unawares. 'Ah well, huh...a few,' he conceded.

'How many of these penises were real and how many were pictures in porn magazines and films?' I shot next.

He looked quite taken aback and wondered how I could so astutely read his mind. I had found my opening. 'Have you ever measured it, your penis I mean, with a ruler or tape?' I persisted.

He confessed that he never had. 'Then how do you know that yours is small? Don't you need to have objective measurements? Penis size is like height, or waist size, you see. One has to measure it. It can't be conjectural.'

'All I know is that, compared to all those pictures and photographs, mine seems really very small,' he managed, finally getting slightly on the defensive. I loved this.

'Has your partner ever told you this?'

'Yes, she has, and it is humiliating,' he admitted sheepishly.

I saved him the embarrassment of asking how his partner knew about such matters. 'Now listen to me,' I continued, 'I've seen thousands of penises in my life, right from the time I was a kid in a hostel. I've seen penises of the young, the not so young, and the old. I've seen Caucasian and other white penises, black penises, oriental yellow penises, and Asian brown penises, not to mention penises of mulattos and other hybrids. I've not just seen them. I have actually measured many of them. So, I ought to know what's normal, what's extra large, and what's small. Right? Do you agree?'

By now, his eyeballs were popping with awe, as if to convey that any man who has seen and measured so many penises must be truly awesome. I badgered on. 'Therefore, now you show me yours and I'll size it up and tell you once for all if you make the grade or not. C'mon here, and lemme take a look.'

Mr Dick stepped forward gingerly, dropped his pants for a dekko, and gave me a 'See, I told you' kind of look. I could barely see the tip of his penis beyond the enormous apron of fat that overhung it. I pulled out a ruler from my drawer, measured whatever penis was visible, and made a note on a pad. I then asked Mr Dick to heave his fatty apron up with both hands and hold it there. A segment of penis that was twice as long as the tip we'd seen earlier came into view. I pulled out my ruler again, measured the penis, and wrote the measurements beside the first one. Dick just stood there holding his belly fat. It was then that I realised that his paunch was so huge that he couldn't even see his own penis. He was oblivious to what I was seeing and measuring. It was like it was happening on someone else's body. Next, I pushed the ruler into the flesh of his pubis, deep up to the bone, and took a third measurement. Then I pulled out the camera from my drawer, captured shots of all three measurements, and showed him the pictures.

'Unless there is some injury or fibrosing disease that causes the penis to lose length, a man's penis size, in both length and girth, usually remains pretty much constant through his adult life,' I explained. However, there is something like a real length and something like an apparent length. The penis is fixed to the pubic bone by a ligament. The real length of the penis is the measurement from this bone to the tip of the penis. When a man puts on weight, the penis gets buried in fat, and much of its length can become invisible. This is called apparent shortening. If the man sheds that fat, or has it removed surgically, that invisible length will become visible again. Therefore, it is important for you to understand that you have not really lost any penile length.'

He swallowed, still skeptical.

I then took him to the window of my office and asked him to peep at the cars parked on the road below. I explained to him how the cars seem to be smaller than they actually are because of the height and distance from which they are being viewed, and that a somewhat analogous phenomenon comes into play when a man looks at his penis in the standing position.

Mr Dick looked fleetingly relieved, and then became grumpy again immediately. It had just sunk into his head that the onus was now on him to shed weight and salvage his buried treasure. The poor guy had probably come to me looking for some shortcut or miracle pill.

'But can't you do a quick operation doc and simultaneously remove all the fat as well as lengthen the penis? I understand that there are operations for penis lengthening and enlargement too.'

Some colloquial phrases from my Mumbai medical college days came to mind. '*Arre, halwaa hai kya?*' (roughly translated, this means something like, 'Do you think this is a piece of cake?'). But I left them unsaid. Instead, I said, 'It's not that simple. The fat that I remove is liable to recur if you are not watchful, and the lengthening operation itself is fraught with complications. Girth enhancement is even more controversial. In general, this kind of surgery is not recommended by experts, especially for the greedy. This is the international consensus at the moment. However, sometimes, we do offer this to the needy ones who are unfortunate to have a really small penis, as opposed to an apparently small one, like in your case.'

Dick looked deflated. All his dreams of becoming a Rasputin overnight had got crushed in an instant. 'Is there no other way?' he persisted.

This was the moment I was waiting for: to explain to him my newest andrological innovation.

'Yes, there are other ways,' I began, with a very serious mien, 'the results with these newer techniques are extraordinary, but there is a slight downside. The penis may not look 100 per cent natural. That, however, might be just a small price to pay for the quite amazing stuff you get in return.'

Mr Dick sat up. Anything which required him to do nothing, but yielded great results, seemed to be instantly appealing to him. 'Tell me all about it, doc. This is probably just the thing I might finally opt for. I guess I have to compromise somewhere or the other, no matter what treatment I choose. A "slight downside" sounds really okay. I don't mind that at all.'

'We have new penis transplant options available to us today. You can choose from between a horse penis, a dog penis, a donkey penis, and a buffalo penis. Other animal penis options haven't been thoroughly researched yet. We're working on some at the moment. But even with just these, you can add many, many inches to your manhood in just a few hours.'

Dick's face lit up like the aurora borealis. I figured that in his mind he was already mounting some beautiful mare that was writhing in the throes of heat. All his studly fantasies were finally about to come true.

I went on to make his sexual sublimations even more sublime.

'Aah, and yes, there's one more unbelievable option that's almost ready now for clinical trials in humans. I've been refining it for the last few years. If this works in the long term, it might turn out to be the most revolutionary medical advance of the millennium. All my hopes of a Nobel Prize in medicine rest on this ingenious one. Would you like to volunteer?'

'Depends, doc. Why not? I just might want to give it a shot. But first tell me more.'

Dick's phallic greed appeared insatiable.

'This new option is an elephant's trunk,' I told him. 'Researchers believe that an elephant's trunk can perform several other amazing functions in addition to just being a copulatory organ. Just think of the mind-boggling possibilities. Apart from stimulating your partner to tumultuous orgasms via every orifice, you could even water plants, pluck fruits off a tree, throttle an enemy, and maybe even deliver your own baby...the possibilities are limitless. It'll even carry shopping bags, push trolleys, and nab pickpockets. Only it hasn't been perfected yet.'

Dick made up his mind faster than I had anticipated and said 'Yes' to the clinical trial. It seemed that he was willing to go to any length for a few inches more.

'That's wonderful!' I said, clapping my hands. 'Let me explain further before I enrol you. The only slight downside with all these operations is that you will have to sacrifice your existing penis. It has to be removed and thrown away or sent to the dissection lab. Only then do we sew on the elephant trunk. Of course, for you I will use an adult male's trunk because you are very size conscious, but even after that there are no guarantees. The transplanted organ might lose its blood supply which comes from your body, die, become black, shrivel up, and might have to be removed surgically. If you are lucky, it sometimes falls off on its own and you can escape the removal operation. Of course, in such sad situations, you will be left with no penis whatsoever. But you could use a strap-on dildo. I have many large models. But you don't look like a man who'll settle for second best. Therefore, you'll have to think carefully and come to a decision only after seriously weighing all the pros and cons.'

Dick's face turned purple first and then a ghostly white. He was breathing heavily and had broken into sweat. He looked like he was going to faint. I turned to my desktop and started checking my email as if nothing was happening. I had seen such responses many times in the past. I wasn't one bit worried about Dick. I only turned when I heard him speak again. He had gotten up, and was now standing.

'Thanks for your time, doc. Research is really amazing. Gimme some time to think about it. Meantime, could you please put me on to a dietician, a good gym, and a personal trainer?'

Any experienced doctor will tell you that we guys in the profession sometimes use unorthodox methods to treat some of our patients. Maybe, but you'll have to admit that these methods work!

I'm waiting for Dick to come back sometime soon with an impressive few inches of salvaged penile pride.

Take Home Message:

For further information on penis lengthening and girth enhancement, the interested reader is referred to *http://www.andrology.com/penisaugmentation.htm*

17

Make Love, Not War

I must confess that, sometimes, in the course of my clinical practice as an andrologist, I feel like an anti-national traitor. India already has more than a billion people, and here I am, helping couples produce more babies to add to this already humungous population figure. Am I doing the right thing? Should I not be catching and sterilising all the men and women who come to me asking for help to produce babies, instead of treating them? What difference does it make if fifteen per cent of the population can't have children? Don't we have enough orphan and destitute children who are in need of nurture and a good home? Why are people obsessed with transmission of their own genetic material?

In certain affluent northern European countries like Germany and Sweden, governments are actually pleading with their citizens to produce more babies because their populations are declining. Couples are being offered special incentives to make babies! Yet, there are not too many takers. And here we are, a billion people wanting to become a zillion. The government exhorts us to 'plan' our families, but nobody cares. In the course of my long career as a clinical andrologist, I have often thought of the Indian *infertility versus population* paradox.

But when I bring up this subject for discussion with peers and colleagues, they call me another kind of traitor instead. A traitor to andrology and reproductive medicine. 'You are going to put all of us out of business if you go on like this, Sudhakar. Your viewpoints are suicidal to our bloody careers, don't you see?' one colleague with thick specs, who specialises in manufacturing twins and triplets, told me. His severe short-sightedness seemed to me to be as much figurative as literal, extending far beyond the merely ophthalmologic.

'You seem preoccupied, doc,' I suddenly heard a voice. 'If this is not a good time, we can always come again later.'

I was jolted out of my mid-day reverie by the young couple in front of me. A seated man had suddenly stood up. Hell, now I was being made to feel like a traitor to my patients! Today was not my day. It seemed more like Traitors Day. I wondered if the Archies and Hallmark guys had thought of that already. And it was only noon yet! I recalled what my wife had told me earlier that morning. She too had alleged that I was a traitor because I didn't drop our daughter to school after she missed the school bus. 'You only think of yourself,' the wife alleged. 'In what way is your surgery more important than my yoga class? If the driver doesn't come one day, I have to become the driver.'

Ultimately, all guys are MCPs, she insinuated.

Meek or termagant, ultimately all women are ball-breakers, I had countered.

Dog's Day was another new concept that came to mind. Again I wondered if the Archies and Hallmark guys had already thought of that too.

Finally I spoke.

'Kindly excuse my preoccupation. I was absorbed with another metaphysical matter. But that's resolved now. Please tell me what I may do for you.'

The gentleman in front of me sat down again. And began, 'Where shall I begin, doc?'

'How about starting with the primary purpose of your visit and then working backwards, if necessary?' I suggested, hoping he'd get the hint right away. That was enough impetus for our man. After that, he was like a dam whose gates had just been opened.

'For the past several months, my wife and I have just been fighting. It's been about two-and-a-half years since we got married, and, right from the beginning, from the wedding night itself, she has been obsessed with just one thing.'

Before I could guess what that one thing was, the chap said, 'Producing babies.'

Shit! My guess had turned out wrong. I let him continue.

'Why are women so competitive when it comes to producing kids, doc? Is it some kind of disease? My wife is always telling me that the so-and-sos have been married only two years and that they already have Monty and Mini, or that this one's gotten pregnant in just six months of marriage, and so on. She also has a lot of inside information about what goes on in other people's bedrooms and about their intimate sex lives. How often they do it. When they do it. What positions they adopt. Which time of the month is best. How many times per day. It's embarrassing for me to learn that my wife is discussing all these things with other people. Aren't these supposed to be intimate and personal things? I'm sure that she tells everyone what we do in our bedroom too, though she denies it vehemently when I confront her. I'm sure all her friends think that she's a fertile goddess and that I'm some kind of sterile wimp in the bedroom. To her, making babies is like a contest she just has to win. But right now, everybody else but her is winning it.' He paused.

'The maternal instinct and yearning in women is a very strong one,' I told him, thinking that the last prize his wife won must've been at a rangoli competition in college. I could understand her need to win another one, especially this one. There's something about rangolis and motherhood. They connect. I plodded him to get on with his tale. I had begun to enjoy it now.

'Yeah doc, but there's a limit to everything. Will it be the end of the world if we don't have kids? We'll try to have them, of course, but is that the sole purpose of our existence? Does everything, from morning to night, have to revolve around this? The other day, she called me up in the office and ordered me to come home right away. When I asked if there was some emergency, she said, "Yes, of course, but why don't you understand, I can't tell you over the phone."

'I was in the midst of some chaos in the office myself, and going home was unthinkable to me. Goddamn it, home was twenty-six kilometres away! When I persisted with wanting to know what the matter was, she started sobbing and screaming on the phone and told me that I didn't care about her and that she plans to call up her father and go to his house right away. I was now really worried. Is there something so serious that she cannot tell me over the phone? Am I being an inconsiderate SOB?'

He paused for breath. Everyone needs oxygen.

'Feeling like a heel, I abruptly put all work matters on hold and charged out of the office. Luckily, the afternoon traffic was not too bad. I kept chewing my nails and honked and snarled at a few pedestrians and autos en route home. My poor baby, I was saying to myself. I hoped that nothing calamitous had befallen her. I would have never forgiven myself if I reached too late and was not there in my wife's hour of need. I was perspiring, breathing hard, and smoking incessantly. The inside of the car was so hazy with smoke that, with the air conditioning on, visibility was blurry. I was coughing and choking moreover. I finally reached home and charged up the stairs, praying to God for the first time in many, many years.'

Interrupting his story now would be really lousy timing, like coitus interruptus, I told myself, and waited for him to resume. This man didn't seem to be running out of words.

'Ten doorbell rings, and there's no answer, doc. When I tried to call my wife's mobile and the home line, there was no answer. Should I call the cops, or ask the neighbours? I started pounding on the door. Still there was no answer. Finally, I realised that I had my house keys right there in my pocket, along with the car keys. With sweaty and shaky fingers, I turned the key and prised the door open. Guess what I saw, doc?'

This guy ought to have been writing thrillers and making movies, not babies, I thought to myself. How could I guess? With this Alfred Hitchcock, anything was possible. My only thought was that so far there wasn't any real andrology discussed.

'I hope it was nothing serious,' was all I could think of.

'You won't believe it, doc. The house was in pitch darkness. All the curtains were drawn. The living area was empty. Petrified, I tiptoed to the bedroom, prepared for the worst. And what do I see?'

He burst out laughing.

My stoic demeanour remained unchanged. I've been around.

'Doc, my wife is absolutely stark raving mad, I tell you. There was soft music playing in the bedroom, the lights were dim, some aromatic candles had been lit, and a small table for two was laid out, with a bottle of champagne and two glasses. I couldn't see the wife anywhere. I had no clue about how to react to all this. My fear had turned to shocked relief, to bewilderment, and now rage. I pushed the bathroom door open and went in to check. My wife was hiding behind the shower curtain, wearing a sheer nightgown and musky perfume. She sprang forward, threw her arms around my neck, and start kissing me passionately. I was surprised to note that I was actually so relieved that I even joined in the fun. My wife then grabbed my hand and slapped a folded piece of paper on my palm. I looked at the paper but didn't have a clue to what it was.'

'My ovulation chart, dude. I have ovulated! Today's the big day man. We just HAVE to do it right here and now. This is our best chance.'

'With that, doc, can you believe it, she peeled off all her pretensions to clothing.'

I observed that this chap had a natural aptitude for crescendos. I didn't want to interrupt his climax.

'I succumbed to the enchantress in her even as I was cursing myself for having left the office so irresponsibly and hating myself for being so weak. I had lost both at work and at home. "Let me take a quick shower first," I mustered. I recalled that in the Housie games I've watched so often at clubs, there always was a Lucky Loser. That day, it was my turn.'

I once again thought of the Archies and Hallmark Guys. 'Loser's Day'!

'This was three months ago, doc, and she still hasn't conceived. That's why we are here. We are fighting with each other every day. Neither feels like making love any more, no matter what. Nonetheless, my wife is desperate to get pregnant at any cost. How can I make love to her, doc, when she's at war with me all the time? We have been seeing specialists for more than a year and have been told that all our tests are completely normal. Some have advised a test tube baby. One doc asked me to undergo an operation. My relatives say that we should try alternative medicine. We don't know whom to follow, what to believe. We are at the end of the road.'

After a detailed talk and a perusal of all their reports, I concluded that theirs was a classical case of overkill. Too much anxiety, too much investigation. I decided that these guys needed a break from all this. I recommended to them that they lay off all plans to have a baby for the next several months and just enjoy themselves and their sex lives all over again like newlyweds. No tests. No treatments. I set them a deadline of six months. 'After six months, if we don't see any progress, we'll get aggressive,' I assured them.

I didn't hear from them for several months after that. I had almost forgotten about them. Then one day, after more than a year, I got a call from Mr Hitchcock*.

'You were absolutely right, doc! My wife's due to deliver in another four months or so. I just thought I should inform you. Thanks so much for everything.'

My Belgian professor's words came to mind. 'Remember one thing Sudhakar,' he had once told me, 'Sometimes, in infertility, doing nothing is everything.'

I couldn't agree more. The Hitchcocks were proof paramount.

Take Home Message:

Infertility is defined as an inability to conceive after one to one-and-a-half years of regular, unprotected sexual intercourse. Only after that period must an infertility

---

*Any pun imagined, not intended

evaluation begin. Unfortunately, many people are unaware of this and seek treatment much sooner. This leads to a lot of unnecessary anxiety, emotional, mental and relationship strains, and needless expenditure. All this can be avoided with proper education. Further information on male infertility is available on *http://www.IndiaInfertility.com*.

18

Men Oh Pause!

'*Male menopause is a lot more fun than female menopause.
With female menopause, you gain weight and get hot flushes.
Male menopause? You get to date young girls and drive
motorcycles.*'

RITA RUDNER
Hollywood Comedienne

[Synonyms: late onset hypogonadism, andropause,
viropause, male climacteric, ADAM, PADAM]

Many who have followed President Bill Clinton's
'sexcapades' or have watched Dev Anand running
around trees at age eighty will readily agree with Rita Rudner.
But how right is she? Do men really suffer a menopause?

It has been long known to scientists that a cock's comb is
a result of circulating testosterone hormone in the blood. One
hundred and fifty years ago, Berthold showed that transplant

of another cock's testis into a castrated cock prevented atrophy of its comb. In 1994, Carl Heller and Gordon Myers described the male menopause. They compared the symptoms with those of the female menopause, and showed the effectiveness of testosterone replacement treatment. Unfortunately, this either went unnoticed, or was suppressed. Men were unwilling to accept the emasculating concept of 'menopause' and such research got hurriedly brushed under the carpet. Men with genuine symptoms suggestive of a probable andropause-like condition were told that 'this is just a mid-life crisis', that everyone goes through it, and that it will pass. Subsequently, testosterone itself came into disrepute as a drug because of its abuse by athletes without proper medical recommendations and guidelines, and there was much hype about its side effects, especially prostate cancer. The whole matter of the andropause and testosterone replacement therapy for its treatment was shelved indefinitely.

It was only after the dramatic results of HRT (Hormone Replacement Therapy) in post-menopausal women became known, that men, not wanting to get left behind looking like their wives' fathers, sat up and began to take notice! Today, there is no denial or controversy.

The andropause, most emphatically, exists.

Unlike in the woman, where there is a sudden cessation of ovarian function and oestrogen production comes to an abrupt standstill, the andropause in the man is characterised by a more gradual decline in the levels of free available testosterone (FAT, or bioavailable testosterone). This testosterone measurement is a bit different from the conventional testosterone estimations that are usually performed at most laboratories, and which are not helpful in the diagnosis of andropause. The sophisticated tests for the diagnosis of andropause are available only at some specialised centres. Unfortunately, neither the andropause nor the tests available for its evaluation are widely known among physicians and some doctors will simply pooh-pooh the very entity of andropause out of sheer ignorance. Awareness on this subject is slowly spreading though, both among medical professionals as well as the laity.

Some of the factors known to contribute to the onset and severity of the andropause are hypothalamic and testis insufficiency, obesity, hormone deficiencies, excessive alcohol consumption, smoking, hypertension, many drugs, unbalanced diets, lack of exercise, poor circulation, stressful lifestyles and psychological problems. A decline in potency at mid-life can be expected in a significant proportion of men since testosterone, the hormone that declines in andropausal men, is also the same hormone that is responsible for sexual drive and libido in human beings of both sexes. Testosterone also has a direct beneficial effect on erections in the human male.

Even in healthy men, it has been found that, by the age of fifty-five, the amount of free testosterone in the blood is significantly lower than it was just ten years earlier. In fact, by age eighty, most males will reach pre-pubertal testosterone levels, that is, their blood testosterone levels will be like that in small boys before adolescence.

At least forty per cent of men between forty and sixty will experience lethargy, lack of energy, decreased work performance, depression, increased irritability, mood swings, reduced enjoyment of life, hot flushes, insomnia, decreased libido, weak orgasms, reduced strength and stamina, weakness, loss of both lean body mass and bone mass (making them susceptible to hip fractures), reduced erectile rigidity, and difficulty in attaining and sustaining erection (impotence).

Sometimes andropause can strike as early as at age thirty-five. This young population of andropausal men is increasing rapidly today, thanks to the trials and tribulations of modern living. However, men with andropause can continue to father children. This is unlike in menopausal women. Nearly all menopausal women are rendered infertile after menopause.

Tips for coping with the changes brought about by the andropause include finding new ways to relieve stress, eating a nutritious, low-fat, high-fibre diet with special food supplements, getting plenty of sleep, exercising regularly, finding supportive groups and sharing, limiting one's consumption of alcohol and caffeine, drinking lots of water, and modifying lifestyle radically. Testosterone replacement therapy must be only administered by very responsible physicians. Even though the newer forms of testosterone are extremely safe and well tolerated, their long-term administration and the monitoring of patients requires expert knowledge and commitment in order to minimise potential complications in some susceptible patient groups.

Testosterone must not be used as a tonic for vague, non-specific complaints, without proper clinical and laboratory corroboration, as it can cause serious side effects, including aggravation of prostate cancer. Patients with proven low serum

FAT (Free Available Testosterone) levels are offered testosterone therapy if they have the other clinical symptoms and signs. Before starting, a complete general check up and some special tests are conducted. These must be repeated at intervals for as long as treatment is continued.

Testosterone is available in oral, injectable, skin patch, cream, gel and implant forms. Doses must be tailored to achieve normal FAT levels and amelioration of symptoms. Significant symptom relief can be expected with treatment. However, all impotence may not respond to testosterone and some more special tests and additional treatment may sometimes be necessary.

So, the next time you see a middle-aged man making a buffoon of himself on the dance floor with a Pretty Young Thing, it might be a good idea to ask him to see his andrologist. After all, sensible ladies his age do see their gynaecologists. Now you know why athletes and other sportsmen are the youngest ones to hang up their boots. They understand reality.

And are you wondering whether it is the andropause that made you buy those ultra-tight black jeans and cowboy boots last week? The ones that hurt your crotch and compelled you to walk with your two feet placed three feet apart?

You can bet that it almost certainly IS andropause! Check yourself out. You'll be thankful for it.

For more information on andropause, the reader is referred to *http://www.andropause.co.in*

19

Late Comers and Marathon Men

A rather grim looking young man came to me recently saying that he had a peculiar problem.

'Relax, no problem is too peculiar for me,' I said, with the smug sagacity that comes naturally to someone who's seen and heard it all. 'Go on.'

'You see doc,' he began, 'My problem is somewhat the opposite of premature ejaculation. I just can't come. Intercourse goes on and on but there's no ejaculation.'

Alfred Lord Tennyson's *The Brook* sprung to mind immediately:

> *For men may come*
> *And men may go*
> *But I go on forever*

Sounds like the story of this man's life, I thought to myself, and wondered if Tennyson had thought of this andrological angle in his famous poem whilst writing it.

I urged the Marathon Man to continue and tell his poem of woe in detail. Having once begun, the guy couldn't stop. He certainly didn't sound like a man who finished anything in a hurry. Finally, I had to gently interrupt him and put two and two together for him myself.

Mr Marathon Man, it transpired, was suffering from a condition known as delayed or retarded ejaculation (RE). RE is defined as a persistent difficulty in achieving ejaculation despite the presence of adequate sexual desire, erection and stimulation. To add to his miseries, his wife and he hadn't made a baby even after four years of marriage.

On the surface, RE might sound like a slogan for Onida TV but often it is more a cause for worrying than for rejoicing. The male goes on for a half hour or more with little sexual pleasure, and constantly worries about when he is going to 'come'. The female usually has already attained orgasm and waits eagerly for the man to finish the remainder of the ritual. She stops lubricating shortly after orgasm and thereafter, the remainder of the sex act is merely a painful formality for her.

In severe cases, the man cannot ejaculate at all. This phenomenon is called anejaculation. We'll talk about this in a while. RE can be both psychological and physical. Psychological causes include anger or resentment towards women, marital conflict, an oppressive upbringing, lack of emotional involvement with partner, fear of commitment, underlying anxiety, fear, depression, and obsessive compulsive disorders. Physical causes include substance abuse (alcohol and drugs), many prescription drugs (antihypertensives and psychotropics), neurological and endocrine illnesses, diabetes, cancer, prostate problems and surgical intervention that affects the ejaculatory apparatus. You see, the list of causes is just as long as the ejaculation time in these guys!

I went on to explain to the Marathon Man that positive reinforcement of operative conditioning associated with masturbation might play a key role in the development of RE. Most men have their first orgasm through masturbation. Many men exert much more pressure during masturbation than they are likely to experience during intercourse. They mistakenly think they need that same pressure to reach coital orgasm. Men can learn to reach orgasm with a partner if they practise stimulation slowly and with much less pressure than usual.

I saw him gulp. He must have definitely thought that I was some kind of mind reader because I noticed him staring at his right palm very symbolically. I could have sworn that I saw guilt on his face. I made a mental note to address that separately.

'When you are suffering from RE,' I continued, 'the trick is to focus on things that are arousing to you. The brain has an amazing way of propelling sexual arousal forward even when the physical stimulation is different or less intense than usual. Teach your partner how to stimulate you in the way you like best.'

The Marathon Man shifted his gaze from his right palm to his left one. Must be ambidextrous, I guessed.

'Good sex can become great sex if subtle nuances, personal preferences and kinks are factored in. You must be in a state of mind that welcomes the sexual sensation your partner is offering you. Check whether you are focusing excessively on giving your partner pleasure. If you are, make sure you don't forget your own needs. Sex is as much about receiving as giving.'

'You're probably right about that, doc,' the Marathon Man said, 'For me it's always been, like, something I do to my wife, not something that we do together, for each other.'

With that, he suddenly developed a glazed, wizened look, which made me think of someone who had long ago sat under a Bodh tree.

'Please continue doc,' he beseeched, 'I am listening very intently.'

That sounded like music to my ears.

'Often, intercourse is begun too soon in the sexual encounter,' I went on. 'Many men with RE believe they'd better start working at it early because they fear that their partner will tire out if the whole experience takes what the partner considers "too long". This leads to missing many an erotic experience that builds arousal. Rushing to intercourse, in essence, short-circuits matters. Going straight to intense genital stimulation numbs what could have been intense pleasure if only it had been built up in graded fashion. Also, give up watching the clock. Many women enjoy a man's taking his time while moving through his sexual responses. Keep in mind, also, that you can stimulate yourself to orgasm while in bed with a partner. The ejaculatory reflex has both central and peripheral neurologic control mechanisms and RE occurs because there is over-control or difficulty in release at one or both levels.'

The Marathon Man couldn't believe that he could get so much for just one consultation. He conspiratorially told me that he's been through many sessions of counselling with several specialists before finally coming to me. I deftly changed the subject.

'Physical causes require separate work-up and treatment, and anejaculation will merit a different approach,' I said. With that I proceeded to tell him some more about other ejaculatory problems.

'In contrast to RE, where there's merely a delay, however inordinate, the entity called anejaculation implies a complete inability to ejaculate. There are many scientific classifications of anejaculation but I'll try and keep it simple. In situational anejaculation, as the term denotes, the man cannot ejaculate in certain situations. A classical example of this is the man who ejaculates normally during sex but cannot, for instance, collect a sample of semen by masturbation during infertility treatment. This is very common. The wife is undergoing treatment and suddenly the infertility specialist pronounces that she has ovulated (released eggs) and that now is a good time to send some sperms up to meet these ova and say hello. The man is asked to produce a sample of semen. Often, a bottle is thrust into his hand and he is directed to a dirty, small toilet. He is expected to lock himself there for a few minutes and come out with a bottle full of sperm! Little wonder that many men have problems doing it. Another situation is somewhat analogous to that discussed in Chapter 17 *(Make Love, Not War)*, where again, it is the wife's ovulation that dictates that a couple should have sex. Only, unlike our protagonist in that chapter, some guys simply can't do it. Not only do many men have problems ejaculating in such situations, many can't even obtain erections sufficient to enable sexual intercourse. That's how stressful and asexual they find the whole context. And then there are some who have never been able to ejaculate in the waking state. These men never discharge semen during masturbation or intercourse. However, they do ejaculate occasionally in their sleep. Luckily, for such cases, cures are easy. We now have machines known as vibroejaculators and electroejaculators, which are very successful at making these guys ejaculate. Success rates with these machines are purported to be almost 100 per cent. These machines are also used to obtain semen samples in men with spinal cord disorders and paraplegias, with similarly good success rates.'

'There are also mechanical causes that can block the sperm conduction passages and make ejaculation totally impossible at all times. And lastly, there are those unfortunates called retrograde ejaculators. In these men, there is semen production and ejaculation, but the semen does not come out through the penis to the outside. Instead, it goes backwards into the urinary bladder, gets mixed with the urine, and gets passed along with it. We're not discussing these last two conditions in detail here but many in this category will require surgical or other intervention for treatment.'

'So what have we learnt here?' I asked the Marathon Man at the end of my sermon, thinking that I had done pretty well for the day.

'Three important lessons, doc,' he replied. '(1) Taking matters in your own hands may not always solve all your problems. (2) Coming 'fashionably late' at bedroom parties is sure to upset your hostess. (3) Some men literally don't know whether they are coming or going.'

The guy turned out to be a lot smarter than I had imagined. Both of us broke into laughter.

20

Non-throbbing Heartthrob

Just a few days ago, a rather cherubic middle-aged man walked into my office. Accompanying him was a considerably younger and attractive woman, who I presumed was the wife. One can usually tell. The 'for better or for worse' part is unmistakable.

'Do you like the Beatles, doc?' Mr Cherub began abruptly, without preamble. This was certainly a new one on me, but I didn't flinch. 'Sure, I grew up with the Beatles,' I returned, concealing my bewilderment rather adroitly.

'Have you heard the song *Yesterday?*' he fired next.

I nodded in the affirmative. Suddenly, Cherub seemed very happy with his choice of doctor. I suspected that if I had said that I hadn't heard of the Beatles or if I had said that I didn't much care for their music, he might have even changed his doctor. He seemed like a man of conviction.

'Well, my story is somewhat like the lyrics of that song, doc,' he began. And then, you are not going to believe this, he burst into song! Can you imagine this? This guy was actually sitting across a doctor's consultation table in the capacity of a patient, and singing a song! The Americans have a word for this. They call it chutzpah. Once I was over the initial alarm, I played along with the singing. I normally ask my patients to calm down, take it easy, and relax. Cherub was doing the same thing with his singing, I reasoned. I thought him to be a pretty cool and original kind of chap with his own unique methodology. I began to feel bad that such a jolly good fellow had developed an andrological problem that necessitated a visit to me. I turned empathetically towards the wife. Her eyeballs had rolled heavenwards, and remained fixed there. Her hands were clutching the armrests of her chair, and her knuckles had turned white. It was quite obvious that she wasn't one bit impressed. I wondered how long she had had this brand of music inflicted on her.

This is what his musical medical history was:

Apparently, until yesterday, all of Mr Cherub's troubles had seemed far away, but now, it looked like they were here to stay. Also, until yesterday, apparently love was an easy game to play, but now Mr Cherub, not being even half the man he used to be, needed a place to hide away.

Unarguably, this was the most musical medical history ever obtained by any doctor in medical history. I wondered if something like this would qualify for a place in the *Guinness Book of World Records*. I've always yearned for a place there. I made a mental note to check this out and push for it before another doctor beat me to it. You see, our medical profession is a fiercely competitive one. The cut-throat mentality begins at the pre-medical level itself. I have to be fast and discreet, I told myself. Adding a Guinness Book to my Limca Book would be quite nice...

I was jolted back into sharp focus by the sound of Cherub's voice. Song sung, he was now speaking. It took me a while to figure the difference between his singing and his talking.

'By now, it must seem pretty clear to you doc that I am suffering from severe erectile dysfunction,' he announced self-diagnostically.

'Any more songs or is this all for today?' was all that I was dying to know. By now, I had even forgotten that this was a consultation in my office. I had the surreal feeling that I was in some nuthouse. Had he at least sung tunefully, I'd have put up with all this, but Cherub's singing was reminiscent of an old HMV gramophone player when voltage fluctuations alternated with power trips. It was unbearable. What made it even more annoying was the fact that he thought himself very mellifluous and sang with a blissful lack of insight.

'How long have you had this problem?' I asked, moving on.

'It's been going on for more than six years now, doc,' the lady finally piped in, logging in her presence when it mattered most. This must be the topic she is most interested in, I deduced. 'Over the past four years, ever since he underwent his bypass operation, our sex life has become zero. Zilch. Zippo. Nada. Cipher. We are more like platonic enemies these days.'

That explains all the discordant music, I thought to myself. But to refer to six years as yesterday seemed a bit euphemistic.

Yester*years* might have been more appropriate. Mr Cherub was certainly in a time warp.

'How did it all begin?' I needed to know.

'Well doc, I am forty-eight now. Things were fine about seven or eight years ago. In fact, at that age I was sexually insatiable and very demanding. My wife thought that I had a one-track mind and naturally didn't share my enthusiasm on the subject. I also never had any problem in the performance department and my wife didn't ever complain. Then suddenly, I noticed a steady decline in my erections. Not only were they not as rigid as before, I also developed sustenance problems. At first I thought it's just one of those passing phases, but it wasn't. It only got worse. Then came my heart attack and I underwent a multiple coronary bypass. I recovered well after the operation but lost erection completely. My wife, whose nickname for me was "heartthrob", says jokingly now that both my heart and my throb are gone.'

I was not at all sure about the 'jokingly' part of it. Again, I turned to look at the wife. It appeared that the only thing in her life that was throbbing right now was her head.

'But why have you lost so much time seeking andrological help?' I asked, 'You could've taken treatment so much earlier.'

'I agree with you, doc. For the first year or so after my bypass, we were devastated and didn't even think about sex. The heart attack was a life and death issue, after all. It was only when life started returning to normal that the need for sex reappeared. But we didn't know where to go. Only recently, someone referred your name to us. In between, I thought I would try Viagra but my doctor warned me that it could be dangerous since I am still on nitrates. So here we are.'

In fact, because impotence (ED) is mostly an arterial disease, and because the arteries to the penis are so narrow, it often precedes heart disease. The incidence of impotence in patients with treated heart disease is seventy-eight per cent for non-smokers and a staggering 94.3 per cent for smokers. The incidence of coronary artery disease among Indians is very high and it is estimated to affect forty-four per cent of those under fifty years of age. It is indeed ironic that despite the magnitude of the problem, few seek help for their condition. Recently, ED (impotence) has been identified as a marker for coronary arterial and cerebrovascular disease. This means that many men who develop ED will go on to develop heart attacks and strokes. In this sense, ED is a useful warning bell since it warns of impending catastrophe. Another clinical triad, in which depression, ED, and vascular disease (high blood pressure, high cholesterol, etc.) often co-exist in the same patient, has also been described recently.

Mr Cherub finally got cured with penile prosthetic implantation surgery. His case is classical and is representative of the plight of millions like him. Heart (and vascular) disease is one of the commonest causes of ED.

Cherub called me recently to tell me that he was writing the lyrics for his new song. 'It's called 'Tomorrow will be even brighter than today', doc,' he told me conspiratorially over the phone, like he was giving me a sneak preview. I was happy for him and congratulated him on his song, but hung up abruptly.

I was afraid he'd start singing over the phone!

Take Home Message:

There is a very close inter-relationship between erectile dysfunction and coronary heart disease. The same disease processes, *viz.* arterial narrowing and cholesterol deposition in the arterial walls, are often responsible for both. In fact, the arteries to the penis are much narrower than the coronary (heart attack) and carotid (stroke) arteries, and get blocked much earlier in the course of progression of the arterial disease. This is why ED is a marker for coronary and other vascular disease. Men with high blood pressure, diabetes, high cholesterol, high lipids, obesity, and smokers, must be on high alert. Physicians treating these conditions in their patients must also discuss with them the risks of developing ED and other vascular disease. When they co-exist, all conditions must be treated simultaneously.

21

High and Dry

The other day my office telephone rang and a gentleman asked to speak with me. 'I have a problem, doc,' he began, 'I'm speaking from Delhi. I cannot come.'

'First tell me what the problem is, then I'll tell you if you need to come to Hyderabad,' I said.

'No, no, doc, you just do not understand, I just cannot come,' he persisted.

'Now, please listen to me, will you? I am *not* asking you to come here. Can you at least tell me what the problem is?' I countered, trying to remain calm.

'What I am trying to say is...doc...my semen does not come out. I just cannot ejaculate,' he concluded, helpfully.

'How long has this been going on?' I inquired.

'All my life, doc,' he cried, 'I have never ejaculated in my whole life. But now that we've been married four years, my wife is desperate to have a baby. That's why I'm calling you.'

The number of husbands who call me because their wives are desperate for one thing or the other is not funny. Unfortunately, there are social, legal, and moral restrictions on the way in which I can mitigate their desperation. Therefore, I only treat the husband.

'Do you ejaculate at least during masturbation?' I asked.

'No, doc, never. I told you, I have never ejaculated in my whole life.'

'Do you at least from time to time ejaculate in your sleep?'

'A little bit only doc, maybe once in a while. But why are you asking me the same thing again and again? I am telling you, I have never ever even once ejaculated in my life during sex, and that ought to tell you something about my case.'

I told him to calm down and that I should be the one getting exasperated, not he. First of all, he is obtaining a professional consultation on the telephone without either an apology or a modicum of thankfulness. Over and above this, he is being argumentative. I told him not to waste my time and that I was going to hang up if he continued like this. I wanted to tell him to call my secretary, obtain an appointment, and show up in person, but softened eventually instead, and continued after he apologised for all inconvenience caused in a *volte face* that is prototypical of his ilk. He uttered about thirteen obeisant *Haan Ji*s in under one minute. I actually counted.

'What about orgasm? Do you reach orgasm during intercourse at least?', I persisted.

'Well doc, I do attain some sort of climax, if you can call it that in the absence of ejaculation,' he said dryly.

'Have you undergone any tests so far?', I needed to know.

'Well, I've got something called the post-ejaculatory urine examination done, though that seems like a bit of a misnomer when I don't ejaculate at all, and my doctor couldn't explain it either.'

I was beginning to like this chap's English, and his ability to turn a glib phrase. It was even more admirable that he could intersperse *Haan Ji* so smoothly everywhere, like the term itself was borrowed from the English. However, I had to remind myself that this was a seminal discussion and not a semantic one. That's one of the downsides to being a doctor. People always expect you to be serious. It's like we guys are some morbid ogres without any sense of humour or other interests in life. Had I commented on this guy's English, or his *Haan Jis*, he would have thought me not serious enough, so I went back to my funereal demeanour. That always impresses patients, even if the subject of discussion is something as pleasurable as multiple orgasms or ultra long-lasting erections. Occupational hazard, some call it. I call it a curse. My mental peregrinations were rudely interrupted by another *Haan Ji*. This was the guy's way of telling me that this is a long distance call. My mind came back at once to the present subject of discussion.

'Yes, indeed, "post-coital" or "post-masturbatory" urine might have been better terms,' I concurred. 'What did the reports show?'

'No sperm in that either, doc, but the lab wasn't sure, and they wanted me to repeat it.'

'Any other tests?'

'Yes, they did something called a TRUS. They inserted some huge horrid probe into my rectum to examine something. It was a most uneasy sensation, I tell you. I was thoroughly disgusted. Anyway, that test too was normal. Now, the doctor wants to do a vasogram. He wants to poke some needles near my testes, inject some dyes, and take some X-rays, but I wanted to check it out with you first.'

'You don't need a vasogram,' I told him categorically, 'It's not going to add any diagnostic value and is needlessly invasive. Besides, even if it is at all necessary, it has to be done in a particular way. I'd like to see you in person, so please make an appointment with my front desk.'

This time he didn't tell me that he couldn't come. His last words on the telephone line were...you've guessed it...'*Haan ji!*'

History-taking disclosed that Mr Haan Ji had no predisposing causes. He had no spinal cord injury, no previous pelvic or retroperitoneal surgery, no diabetes, infections or neurologic disease, and no history of drug use or injury. He thought that he had undergone some operation on the urinary system during his childhood but couldn't tell me details. A psychosexual screening was performed and found to be quite normal. For all other practical purposes, the couple seemed to be very happily married.

Finally, as is quite common in medical practice, the bombastic diagnosis of 'idiopathic (of unknown cause) anejaculation' was made. Mr Haan Ji's problem was solved a few months later using a machine known as the electroejaculator. The electroejaculator allows the application of an electric current trans-rectally to the ejaculatory apparatus. This electrical stimulation causes ejaculation. Newer machines assure nearly 100 per cent success rates. The semen is collected and inseminated into the wife at the time of ovulation. Mr Haan Ji from Delhi now has a bonny baby and his wife seems unlikely to hassle him at least for some time!

Ejaculatory disturbances constitute a complex group of common conditions which are sometimes very difficult to treat. Anejaculation is a condition where there is no ejaculation at all during sexual intercourse. Sometimes, the anejaculation is total, that is, the man does not ejaculate under any circumstances, not even in his sleep. Obstructive causes are usually cured by surgery. Others will require vibrator therapy or the electroejaculator, with excellent results.

Mr Haan Ji was passing through Hyderabad recently and called me. 'Doc, can I call you Dr Nokia?' he asked.

I wondered what it was this time, and asked what that meant.

'Doc, you're always connecting people, isn't it? So tell me, can I call you Dr Nokia?'

What could I say? '*Haan Ji,*' I replied.

For further information on anejaculation, please visit *http://www.anejaculation.com*

22

Reel Life and Real Life

To many Indians, reel life is real life. Films have a profound impact on the beliefs and value systems of the people of India. What the common man sees on the screen, he believes to be true, and tries to emulate. The vast majority of films churned out by our prolific multi-lingual film industry are family dramas in which the romantic, inter-personal relationships between men and women constitute the central theme. What is depicted on celluloid, therefore, could end up laying the moral, sexual and gender codes for millions and millions of impressionable people. In fact, cinematic sex education is perhaps the only form of sex education that most of our people ever receive. That is, if you can call imparting of all the wrong kinds of information 'education' at all.

This is dangerous.

Film-making is thus a serious responsibility and our film makers should not only be conscientious of their own accord, they should also be held accountable for the kind of stuff that they peddle in their films. There is no doubt that India boasts some really world class talent in many different areas of film-making. But the handful of films that are made by this esoteric lobby are viewed only by the literati. The overwhelming majority of India is fed, and thrives on, balderdash.

It is dangerous for us to suppose that people flock our theatres for a few hours of cheap, mindless entertainment, and that they forget what they've seen the minute the film is over and they walk out of the cinema hall. This is not true at all. People believe what they see. And the more young and impressionable the mind, the more seriously does it believe it.

Let us now take a look at some of the dangerous stereotypes that are depicted in our films.

The protagonist male: Commonly known by the absurd title of 'hero', this man is really made to act and behave like one. In the classic potboiler, everything that he does is heroic. If it is college, even if he looks fifty, he always tops the university. If it is sport, he is always first in all events. If it is a fight, he always wins, even if he is pitted against an army of baddies. If it is romance, he always gets the most attractive girl, pipping several other eligibles and wealthy goons to the post. If it is about being a brother, he is exemplary. No one in the world can be a sibling like him. If it is about being a son, he is even better, especially in relation to his mother. She is his everything, and *vice versa*. The term *khandaan ka chiraag* (lamp/light of the family) is not to be taken lightly. The mother's every wish is the hero's command. Even his paycheck is handed to the mother first. And if the father were to reprimand him for any one of several inanities he is constantly shown performing on screen, *Maa*, *Amma* or *Mummy* is sure to support her *Munna* or *Kanna*, if not overtly, at least covertly. This includes playing Cupid in the son's usually exciting love life, which is filled with college picnics, songs, and dances. No woman can ever take the place of the mother in this man's life. To make matters even more ridiculous, the mother is generally shown wearing white, the symbol of purity or widowhood, and is usually a devout lady who cries a lot, visits places of worship and offers prayers regularly, and is either always ill herself, or is tending to the sick and infirm.

This type of mother and son relationship constitutes the gold standard for a nation of one billion people. So where does another woman fit into the hero's life? Read on.

The protagonist female: is also known as the 'heroine', but this is merely a mock title. As we have seen already, the real heroine in every Indian film is the boy's mother. This second class citizen (the mock heroine) is introduced to the viewers in one of several ways. If not as a college student, she is at the very least shown singing or dancing on a stage or in a park in the opening scene. Alternatively, she is shown to be the sole bread winner in a family riddled with tragedies. No matter what the background though, her dance and music skills are usually matchless. If in college, she is usually also first in class and the leader of a large group of servile and sycophantic friends. Many bad guys from the aristocracy try to woo her but she dismisses them all with curse words like *badtameez, neech, kameene, kutte, besharam*, et cetera, and asks them whether they have a mother and a sister at home or not. That is, until the hero arrives, whereupon she blushes and eventually acquiesces to his advances after some initial reluctance and a few songs, and does not call him all these bad names. Though she dances half-naked in the rain, she is actually a pristine, pre-marital touch-me-not. However, occasionally she succumbs to our hero's considerable charms, gets pregnant, and begets twins or triplets after just one night of frolic. (For some reason, to andrology's bad luck, infertility never seems to be a health issue in Indian cinema. TB, abstruse cancers and heart attacks rule the roost there.) Immediately, her attire and demeanour change in a stunning turnabout, and she is shown with head covered, touching her mother-in-law's feet repeatedly. Her hitherto untapped culinary, maternal and house-keeping skills suddenly come to the fore. Every once in a while, she is shown in bed with her husband. As usual, he is desperate to make love, but the mother-in-law's medicines or the children's homework are always more important for her. This, of course, only happens if her husband hasn't died by now already, leaving the heroine also in white to keep her mother-in-law colour co-ordinated company.

This is just some of the garbage that our children grow up on. Only they don't think or know it is garbage, and that's the dangerous part. The new millennium and the electronic invasion have only changed these old trite prototypes somewhat. Nothing like this ever really happens in the lives of any Indian, yet the vast majority of Indian film goers have only have such role models and scenarios to emulate.

At the other end of the spectrum, our people are watching western soaps on the small screen. Here, most of the women are clad in bikinis or their equivalents, boast a minimum bust size of thirty-eight, and have grandmoms who use more makeup than even they do. The men all have six-pack abdomens and everyone is having an affair with everyone else. Sixty-year-old ladies sleep with twenty-five-year-old men and vice versa. This lasts for a few scenes after which they all change partners, divorce, and re-marry. Drugs, alcohol, discotheques, fast cars, airports, and swanky restaurants with overdoses of champagne complete the picture.

To the vast multitude of impressionable masses who are forever looking for role models, cinema can become a powerful influence. No matter what the film-makers may say in order to defend what they are providing to the people in the name of entertainment, I am of the personal conviction that such depictions mostly do more harm than good.

Recently, I asked my wife, 'Aati kya Khandala?' She said, 'Sorry. Don't you know, the children have exams. Also, your mother's arriving tomorrow.'

See what I mean? It's exactly like in the movies.

Take Home Message:

Probably '*Don't take home* everything you see on celluloid!'

23

The New Millennium Woman

Recently, a gargantuan Man Mountain (MM) steamrolled into my office. In tow, was a petite, *purdah*-clad woman molehill. I waved them in and gestured for them to sit down. Yet, both remained standing. When I looked quizzically at them, the lady explained that the chair offered was too small for her husband. He was over six feet tall and weighed about 320 lbs. The other chair was capaciously adequate for the lady though, but yet she chose to remain standing, seemingly in deference to his 'highness'. I apologised profusely and promised to order some XXL chairs soon. This was the first time ever in my career that the need for one had been experienced. Ms Petite said it was all right and that they were used to this. Few places had chairs large enough to accommodate her husband, she said. I realised then that she was the interpreter. The man, it appeared, was from another land, and understood only one language (any pun entirely imagined). He was extremely unhappy to stand and stared at me belligerently throughout the remainder of the consultation.

'Yes ma'am,' I began, 'What may I do for you?'

'Well...' the lady hesitated, 'my husband has a-an-andrology problem.'

I was tempted to tell her that clinics with boards announcing that they are andrology centres normally see only andrology problems and don't treat brain tumours, etc., but since anatomical transposition is not unknown in some humans, and because I didn't want to confuse or offend her, I let that pass.

'What andrological problem?' I goaded instead.

'He...he can't d-do that...thing, doctor. Just can...not. Also we're t-trying to...to have a b-baby,' she stuttered. 'We have been m-mar...ried for one-and-a-half years.'

'How will you have a baby if he can't do it?' I asked, wondering if she had any aspirations towards immaculate conception. 'No, doctor,' she said. 'Can't do it is now. Can't have baby is beforehand. I am his third wife.'

I'd been through such awkward encounters before and didn't want to embarrass Ms Petite any further. I requested her to step out of my office and sit in the waiting room for a moment. The instant she left the room, I swung with gusto into andrological sign language. This is the one universal language that all men understand, and especially MM, I was willing to bet.

Using a skilled combination of some practised gesticulation and rebuses, I had his entire medical history unravelled in a few minutes without uttering a word. Yet he was unimpressed. Macho guy, I thought to myself. Either that or imbecile as hell.

A physical examination on MM revealed that he had the genital size of a ten-year-old boy and pre-pubertal blood testosterone levels. He was unable to even furnish a sample of semen for analysis.

MM had told this third wife that he left his first two wives because they couldn't bear him children in spite of a normal sex life with him. This could not be true. With penis and testes that small, it was extremely unlikely that he had had sex with his earlier wives. He was lying. Also, he had never undergone any previous examination or tests for infertility. Now he was blaming Ms Petite for not being able to do it for him! I wondered how he agreed to come to my office in the first place. Either he must think that doctors are stupid or, that petite lady must be only deceptively meek, I concluded. She might have been the one who tricked him into visiting me.

'So what's new?' I thought to myself. I see cases like these quite commonly. It is quite sad to note how women are blamed for all sexual problems among couples even today when all scientific studies indicate otherwise. Today, it is very well known that fifty per cent of all childlessness is male factor related. We also know that a woman cannot be responsible for a man's impotence unless the man finds her extremely unattractive, or the woman has the track record of Lorena Bobbitt. It seems to be in the interest of some societies and cultures to perpetrate falsehoods about women. What the perpetrators don't realise is that, unfortunately, this is not going to solve the problem. It only delays the inevitable and makes matters worse.

In some ancient cultures it was acceptable for men to hang their wives if they failed to produce offspring. In Regency England a man could publicly denounce his wife if she didn't beget an heir. Queen Mary of England was referred to disparagingly as 'The Barren Queen'. Henry VIII went through several wives in quest of a son. Louis XVI, king of France and spouse of the sensual Marie Antoinette, suffered from infertility. Still, for years the peoples of France angrily blamed the 'Austrian whore' for not producing an heir and instructed her to 'properly perform' her duties. Closer home, India is world famous for infertility related bride burning. The list is endless.

Modern day infertile women are forced to suffer some of the same indignities that women throughout history have been forced to endure, and Ms Petite seemed no exception.

With andrologic treatment, MM showed a slight increase in the size of the penis, and was able to have some kind of sexual intercourse (for the first time) but he would never sire a child. His testes were unresponsive to all treatment and would never produce sperms.

Approximately fifteen to twenty per cent of all couples are infertile, that is, childless. In nearly half of these, it is the male factor that is responsible for the wife's inability to conceive. This means that 7.5 to ten per cent of men are infertile.

Even in the ironical Indian context of one billion people, that makes male infertility a very serious issue.

It's about time that men woke up to this reality. The sexually liberated, economically independent woman is already here. With a pick of both available men and mind-blowing gizmos, she doesn't need an MCP husband for sexual gratification. Moreover, she can just walk in to a sperm bank with her gold card and eugenically choose between the sperm equivalents of a Schwarzenegger or an Einstein if she wants a baby.

A sad end to male chauvinism, perhaps, but a good beginning for female emancipation and infertility in general.

Like Shobhaa Dé had prophesied, the women's millennium has indeed begun.

Take Home Message:

If, throughout history, and until the present time, women have been wrongly blamed for all sexual problems among couples, scientific ignorance and male chauvinism are only partly to blame. In a country like India, where docility is considered the ultimate feminine virtue, women are often trying to score martyrdom points by being silent spectators to their own oppression. This is like some kind of sexual *sati*, and must be abolished.

For further information on infertility, the interested reader is referred to *http://www.andrology.co.in* or *http://www.indiainfertility.com*

24

Stale Mates

One of the nicest fringe benefits of having selected the sub-specialty of andrology as a career is that it makes for great party talk. Even the most inept and inarticulate social conversationalist can find an easy opening line with which to start talking to me. You see, sex is everybody's favourite subject. Nobody wants to talk about morbid conditions like heart attacks, epileptic attacks, paralytic attacks and stuff with doctors, but sex...now, that's a different thing! Besides, many guys are self-proclaimed authorities on the subject of sex too, and, since I'm always willing to learn from the maestros, they find in me a willing victim. Also, it helps people if they say hello to me and are seen talking to me at parties. It serves as the perfect decoy. The conclusion drawn by others when they see someone in animated conversation with me is that this guy can't be my patient, because, if he was a patient, he'd have been too embarrassed to meet me and would have avoided me instead. Anyway, now word has got around about this phenomenon, and nowadays it is in fact my patients who make it a point to come up to me early in the evening to say hello. They feel that this way they'll be above suspicion. I don't complain or pass judgement on all this. I am happy either way because, patient or no patient, I get to meet and talk to a lot of interesting people, both during and outside of working hours.

At a recent party, one such sex pundit strode up to me. Clutched in his right fist was what seemed like his fifth 'large'. Nestled between his left index and middle fingers was a vile smelling Havana. He swaggered up to me with gregariousness oozing from every pore of his being. I braced myself for the oncoming onslaught.

'Howdy, doc!' he began, his left hand slapping my right shoulder hard. He didn't notice the cigar ash that immediately fell on my right shoe. He didn't notice the whisky–soda that fell on my left shoe either. He was just too full of himself to care.

Our man Flint was in a pontific mood. 'I'm telling you doc, all marriages, sooner or later, end in a stalemate. It's like a mix of both. Win-win and lose-lose. More of the latter I suspect though. Finally, even the mate becomes stale.' He guffawed at his own humour and continued, 'By this time, the electricity between man and wife is long gone. The thrill of just a touch or a look that we used to experience in our younger years becomes history. Sex becomes a perfunctory duty and a chore that both parties would rather not engage in. My wife and I have talked a lot about this, doc, and have agreed that we would like to work at obtaining a solution to this within the context of monogamy only. Surreptitious affairs, wife swapping, and open marriage are not for us. We'd rather work on our own marriage.'

Suddenly, I became aware that I was nodding metronomically in response to this soliloquy and was now standing with my back to a wall, approximately fifteen feet away from where this assault began. To my luck, the wall had a large open window. I made a mental note of this emergency exit. I had a feeling that I might need it soon.

'I've done a lot of reading on this subject, doc,' Flint went on, with authority. We've tried everything, well nearly. You see, I'm almost fifty-five now, and my wife isn't much younger. Surely, it's too much to expect us to recreate our wedding night and feed each other cherries, for God's sake! Yet, this is what one of your colleagues, a famous sexologist, has advised us to do.'

I let that pass, and waited for him to continue. He didn't disappoint.

'I believe that even eighty-year-old Americans do this to keep their juices flowing. These guys are crazy, I tell you. As it is my wife says that we must just give up sex because it is so much simpler. She prefers instead to lock herself up in the puja room for several hours.'

I didn't blame her. I would have done the same thing too if I was a woman and being in the bedroom with Flint was the alternative. Flint turned briefly to signal for another drink and I quickly seized the opportunity to pull out the hanky from my pocket and wipe his salivary spray off my face with it. Shortly, his fuel arrived, and he was ready once again for propulsion.

'Aah, where was I? Yess-sss! And then there was this other freaked out therapist who told us to buy some perfumed oils and give each other sensuous massages. He went on to say that throughout the massage we should both mutter naughty, erotic, sexy nothings to one another. When I told my wife all this, she thought I'd gone crazy, and advised me to see a shrink. Her pujas became longer after that.'

My only thought was that these guys would require a considerable amount of oil to cover each other's bodies. I wondered if the stuff was very expensive. Fleetingly, I tried to visualise Mr and Mrs Flint, naked in bed, and slathering one another with oil. A shudder passed down my spine.

But Flint had other plans for me. 'Do you think there's something wrong with me, doc?' he asked rhetorically, 'Why does my wife want me to see a shrink? I assure you, I'm not impotent. I get damn good erections at all other times — especially when I'm alone in the bathroom with myself — EXCEPT when I am trying to have sex with my wife. I tell you doc, this is a serious problem and you must write about it in your columns. I'm certain that this happens in many marriages.'

Just then Flint gestured to the bartender hypnotically, like Mandrake the magician, and a full glass of whisky-soda appeared in his hand from nowhere. I was impressed. Flint's voice jolted me back to the reality of the present.

'What doc? You are not saying anything. I'm the only one doing the talking,' he accused, perspicaciously.

I was quick to seize this rare privilege to squeeze in a few words sideways. I was sure that this favour was not bestowed upon too many people. 'What you say is very poignant indeed,' I reassured him, 'Why don't we discuss it over dinner?'

Mandrake seemed unhappy to relinquish his strangleholds on either me or his drink, but reluctantly agreed after fixing himself one more slugger for the table. By now, we also noticed that most people were leaving.

'So tell me doc,' he pushed.

I told him that human sexuality, both in the male as well as in the female, changes with advancing age, or at least, it should. And that trying to recapture the sexuality of one's twenties in one's fifties is quite absurd. And that one should embrace a new sexuality that is age appropriate.

Just then, Narda (isn't that Mandrake's beloved?) made her appearance out of thin air, just like his drink. Only, this time it was Termagant Narda. 'Oh darling, as usual you are the only one who is still drinking and hasn't eaten,' she uttered ominously.

I understood instantaneously that my friend's term 'stalemate' was the greatest euphemism of all time. And that his term 'win-win' was pure delusion.

This was a one hundred per cent 'lose-lose', 'checkmate' situation. And poor Flint was talking about mating! Better get out of here fast, my antennae told me.

I gestured discreetly to the valet for my car and vanished into thin air.

Take Home Message:

It is true that human sexuality in both sexes changes with age. It is now known that human beings are sexually active until very ripe old age, even in their eighties and nineties. This is nothing to be embarrassed or ashamed about. Geriatric sexuality is very real. Even the aged need love, and sex is but one avenue for its expression. Hence, one should try to embrace an age-appropriate sexuality. Many resources are available on this subject.

25

Deep Purple

It was a Sunday afternoon, I recall, and we had had some friends over with their kids for a beer-n-brunch at our home. This is just my kind of Sunday afternoon, because it gives me an opportunity to indulge in all three of my favourite hobbies: music, photography and bartending. I had taken a lot of trouble to set things up and was all charged.

Firstly, I had pulled out all our favourite CDs, and loaded five of the most popular ones into the multi-CD changer. It was the pre-MP3, pre-iPod era, and this was considered pretty high-tech: to be able to play five CDs at one time in shuffle mode.

Next, I pulled out my Canon SLR camera with all its interchangeable lenses, loaded Kodak 64 film, and mounted it on a tripod. We were all young parents then, and were quite enthusiastic about taking pictures of our children. And our circle of friends was not short on kids. Even the least fertile couples amongst us had at least two children. All our friends would always ask me to take pictures of their kids, and I'd always oblige. Since most people look fairly nice when they are kids, it was also an aesthetic experience. I'd enlarge the pictures and gift it to them on their birthdays and all that. Of course, now that the kids have all grown up, it is a completely different experience. Luckily, with digital cameras, you can easily delete pictures.

The bar was fully organised too. I had prepared a spicy Hyderabadi Bloody Mary in enormous volumes, shoved several bottles of beer into the chiller, and threw in a punch for the non-drinkers and kids. Twenty kilos of extra ice had been ordered. It was going to be a cool, hot summer's day.

Meantime, the waft of succulent *kebabs* had started emanating from the kitchen. We were all set to receive our guests.

A little while later, after the second round of drinks, when the party was in full swing and we were tapping our feet to the beat of Foreigner's *Urgent*, the maid announced that there was a phone call for me. There was some lady on the line who said that her matter was urgent, and that it was an emergency.

I was sure that there was some mistake somewhere. There are almost no emergencies in andrology. Well, actually, that's not altogether true. Thanks to Lorena Bobbitt and some penile injection enthusiasts, we do have some nowadays. But they are not very common. I asked the maid to check out if the call was for my wife because my paediatrician wife is Dr Krishnamurti too, and I thought that the caller must be one of her patient's mothers who wanted to discuss a child's illness with her.

A few moments later, the maid came back to say that the call was not for my wife but for me and that the lady was getting a bit hysterical. Thankfully, it was the pre-mobile era, mind you, or this chick would have caught me in the loo even, I'm certain. She sounded that desperate. Finally, I took the call.

'Thank God, doc! You really had me worried. I thought you were out of town or that you were avoiding my call. We need to see you right now! There's been an accident. My husband's been badly hurt. Can you come home immediately, please?'

The lady was an acquaintance so I had to be a bit tactful. The cut and dry professional approach doesn't work with friends and relatives. They need to be handled with kid's gloves, and plenty of TLC.

'You'll probably need to go to trauma care,' I said, hoping that the poor guy had not sustained a serious head injury or broken a limb. 'I could call the emergency officer at the hospital and put him on alert. I know those chaps there. You go there right now and I'll see you there in fifteen minutes. At least all the first aid stuff and splinting and bandaging will be taken care of by then.'

The lady was getting exasperated and annoyed now. 'Doc, I have not rung you up for social support as a doctor's friend. My husband's accident is andrological. That's the reason why I have called you. He has injured his penis badly. It's all swollen up and looks like an overripe brinjal. I am really scared. What should we do? He is in a state of shock and I can't even tell anyone else in the house about this. Only my in-laws are here now. How can I even *think* of telling them something like this? If I know them, they're sure to blame me even for this. They're always blaming me for anything and everything.'

Experienced old fox that I was, I could gauge the situation accurately now. Some Sharon Stone kind of sexcapade seems to have been attempted, and had misfired. I was trying to guess what it might be.

'I can't even take him to the hospital you have suggested, doc. Everyone knows us there. It's so embarrassing. Can you see him somewhere more discreet?'

'Yeah sure,' I replied, and gave her the address of another place nearby. 'I'll see you there in fifteen minutes.'

Luckily, I hadn't been drinking and, it being a Sunday, was able to leave for the hospital immediately. I reached there before they did. I figured that these guys were still trying to get past the inquisitive parents. I wondered what yarn they were spinning to them. It certainly was a dicey situation.

After what seemed like an eternity, a car screeched into casualty. This is one thing I can never understand about India and Indians. They are late even for emergencies! I was hoping that the poor guy's *baingan* had not become *baghaara*, or *bhartha*, by now. I rushed him to the examination room after giving him a shot of potent analgesic. He dozed off in no time.

Examination revealed that the penis had really swollen up enormously and had become a boggy, spindle-shaped mass. A distinct rent was palpable along the shaft. This was a classical case of what is known as a fracture of the penis.

I applied a dressing to the aubergine organ and stepped out to discuss the matter with the wife. She seemed calmer now. I was hoping it was because of my reassuring presence.

'Can you please tell me in a nutshell what happened, just so that I get an idea? You don't have to tell me any details that you might find embarrassing.'

'Thanks for that, doc. It is pretty straightforward actually. My husband's been bringing home a lot of porn magazines and XXX videos lately, and wants to try out all those acrobatic positions depicted therein. When I tell him that those are all fake and trick photography, he tells me that I don't know anything. So I just indulge him. What else to do? Today, he wanted to do it in the bath tub. "Sunday Special", he called it. I had oil in my hair and had a face pack on, but he didn't care. While we were trying to manoeuvre ourselves into some acrobatic position, he slipped on soap suds and fell. He had a full erection at the time of falling and sustained a direct injury to the penis. I heard a distinct cracking sound too. Not sure if I was just imagining it. Immediately, he cried out in pain and buckled up. Within minutes, the penis had swollen up enormously. Luckily, there's a fridge in our bedroom so I was able to make a quick ice pack and apply it. Then I called you.'

It has been my experience that women are always better at providing andrological histories than men. I guess it's easier for them. Tell the truth and finish it off. There are no macho issues involved.

I explained to the lady that immediate surgery would be the best option for her husband although there is a school of thought that believes in waiting and watching. With the latter approach, I explained to her, recovery time is much greater/more, the swelling lasts much longer, scarring may occur, and the rent in the 'fracture' site doesn't get closed properly. Aesthetic appearances are also much better with immediate operation, recovery is faster, and sexual intercourse can be resumed much earlier.

That last bit seemed to impress her. 'Let's operate, doc. How soon can we do it?'

Two days later, Mr Deep Purple left the hospital, looking quite fit. I didn't hear from them for some time. Usually, no news is good news.

A few months later, I met them at a mall and made polite conversation. 'Is everything all right?' I inquired.

'Depends on how you define 'all right', doc,' said the wife. 'He's gone and bought four anti-skid mats for our bathroom now.'

Take Home Message:

A fracture of the penis occurs when the erect penis is forcibly bent downwards. It is not uncommon and usually occurs due to sexual accidents. Minor fractures with minimal bleeding and swelling can be treated expectantly, but more serious injuries with severe swelling will fare better with early operation. The results of surgery are very good when performed at centres of excellence.

26

Too Hot to Handle

Some years ago, a middle-aged couple came to see me. The husband and wife must have both been in their mid-thirties. Both looked apathetic and listless. I couldn't understand why anyone looking like that would voluntarily seek andrological consultation. You see, andrology is a quality of life (QOL) specialty area in medicine. Those who don't have any interest in life and living in the first place are hardly likely to care much about its quality. Hence, andrology didn't seem at all to fit in with this couple's demeanour.

I thought that these people had made a mistake somewhere. They looked more like lambs being led to a slaughterhouse than like my usual patients. I was almost tempted to tell them that mine is not an intensive care unit or a mortuary, so that they would realise their blunder and go away. To add to my bewilderment, the man was carrying an enormous suitcase. I suspected that he might have even paid excess baggage for it, that's how awesome it looked. I was dying to know what it contained. He probably thought that I was a cardio-thoracic surgeon and had brought along my fees for a coronary bypass operation or something, I figured, using deductive logic.

The mystery was getting deeper and deeper.

Sure, hospitals and clinics are admittedly depressing places and nobody goes there unless it is inevitable. But even at hospitals, such sad looking guys are not an everyday sight. Something was seriously wrong here, I told myself. I was keen to find out what the matter was.

Even though I asked them several times to sit down, the Despondents chose to remain standing. Again, I got the distinct impression that they had regretted coming here. It appeared that a part of them was contemplating turning around and bolting through the door.

Eventually, after what seemed like an eternity, they made up their minds to stay and sat down abruptly. I stared at the ceiling, and waited. Anything happens in this world, I told myself. Only, here it was happening to me.

'We have given up hope, doctor,' the husband finally uttered.

What a way to start! It was certainly not very flattering to me. I wanted to ask them what the point in seeing me was if they had already lost all hope, but I desisted, not wanting to further beleaguer them.

'Can we at least discuss the problem before jumping to hasty conclusions?' I recommended.

I expected him to tell me about the heart attack he had suffered and about the coronary bypass operation he wanted me to perform.

'Well, doctor, let me summarise it for you,' the wife butted in. 'We've been trying to have a baby for six years now, right from the time we got married. For the first four years, we tried diligently, but to no avail. Then we started seeing doctors. Over the past two years, we've visited several and have had eight attempts at IUI (intra-uterine insemination) and three attempts at IVF (in vitro fertilisation — test tube baby). As you can see, they have all been failures. We're tired of scans, semen analyses, injections and medicines. We've spent lots of money, and both of us, being working people, have lost a lot of leave and pay too. We just want to know whether to give up hope altogether or whether it makes sense for us to continue to try. Just tell us bluntly, doctor. My husband has reached a stage where he now can't even have sex or collect a sample of semen on the desired date any more. How much semen they've taken out of my poor baby!'

'At least he's not going to get a heart attack in my office and die right here and now,' I thought to myself, with a sigh of relief. Semen loss and infertility are easy.

'I see what you mean,' I said, understandingly.

Mr Despondent then opened his enormous suitcase and pulled out several massive files. No money there, I noticed. It was an effort for him to lift the thick files and place them on the desk. I went through the pile one by one. The poor man must have undergone nearly two hundred semen analyses. I couldn't help thinking that he might have probably had a better chance of fathering a child if he had inseminated all that semen into his wife rather than surrender it meekly to the lab technician.

When I finished studying the files' voluminous contents, I noticed to my horror that the man hadn't been physically examined by a doctor even once in all these years! It was the wife on whom all examinations and tests had been done. The man was simply handing over semen samples to the fertility centre whenever required. To me, all this seemed less like human husbanding and more like animal husbandry. I couldn't believe it! This was supposed to be the best centre in their town. But I didn't say anything. No point rubbing it in, I thought. They were feeling lousy enough already.

I studied his papers for the next several minutes and then did what I usually do when the facts are overwhelming. I start from the very beginning. I requested the wife to step out for a few minutes saying that I wanted to examine the gentleman. I have never understood the absurd logic behind this strangely Indian medical custom. This couple has been trying to make a baby for six years now, yet I'm asking the lady to leave the room now in the interest of modesty! Corny, but that's how it is usually done in this part of the world. The wife left the room hastily too, with head bowed down in a classical display of Indian feminine hypocrisy. It was almost like she was saying, 'if the lights are on, I'm out; if the lights are out, I'm on'.

The Indian woman, it appears, is a creature of the night, like Laura Brannigan.

A simple physical examination of the man revealed what a second year medical student would have picked up in two minutes flat — a very large left varicocele! The varicocele is the commonest cause of male infertility and yet, two years and hundreds of tests later, it had been completely missed and remained undiagnosed in Mr Despondent's case! What could I say!?

'What's the matter, doc?' Mr Despondent asked, staring down possessively at his unmentionables as I was examining them. Not too many had handled these parts of his body earlier, I guessed. When I finally pronounced that he has a varicocele, he wanted to know everything about it. I asked him to get dressed and call the wife in. No point in having to repeat myself.

I told Despondent that nature has intentionally placed the testes (testicles) outside the body. This is because the core of the human body is hot and, if the testes remain inside there, they cannot produce sperms. The testes need a lower (cooler) temperature in order to produce sperms. By placing the testes outside the body, it is possible to reduce the temperature by three to five degrees Celsius. This is why humans and some mammals have their testes outside their bodies, I explained, and told them how the testes travel all the way from near the kidneys to their final destination in the scrotum, just for this purpose.

'Yes, yes, doctor, now I have understood everything. I have seen testicles hanging out and bouncing up and down in dogs and horses also. Am I right?'

'Absolutely,' I said, thinking him to be rather astutely observant. I continued.

'However, sometimes the veins which carry blood away from the testes back to the heart become long and large. This is known as a varicocele, a condition quite analogous to varicose veins in the leg. When this happens, the blood cannot flow up against gravity efficiently and, in fact, hot blood from inside the body begins to flow backwards into the testes instead.'

'Oh, I see,' said Mr Despondent. 'This means that the testes becomes very hot and cannot produce sperms properly, just like how we cannot work properly in the office without air conditioning. Am I right, doctor?'

I nodded and continued. This man was a lot more brilliant than I had imagined.

'Varicoceles occur in as many as thirty-five per cent of men with primary infertility (inability to father first child) and in as many as seventy to eighty per cent of those with secondary infertility (inability to father subsequent children). Male infertility accounts for nearly fifty per cent of all infertility. While it is true that not all varicoceles cause infertility, many studies (including those by the World Health Organization) have shown that in infertile men with this condition, there is impairment in sperm counts and motility, reduction in testis size and function, and abnormalities in sex hormone levels in the blood. Diagnosis is by clinical examination and scrotal doppler studies. The best treatment method is microsurgery. Conventional surgery, optical loupe surgery, and laparoscopy do not offer the same success rates. Microsurgery can produce successes in eighty per cent of cases and can result in pregnancies in up to sixty per cent.'

Since Mr Despondent had tried every conceivable medicine for conceiving, I unhesitatingly advised him to undergo a microsurgical varicocelectomy operation after conducting a few perfunctory tests. I was the pioneer of this kind of surgery in India and had a large experience, I told them, by way of sales pitch.

'We know doc,' they chorused. I didn't want to embarrass myself by asking them why they hadn't come to me much earlier in the first place then.

The operation was performed under spinal anaesthesia one fine morning, and Mr Despondent left the hospital the same evening.

Eighteen months after microsurgical operation, the Despondents became the proud parents of a beautiful baby girl. It was time to change their name now. Taking a cue from my lawyer friends, I renamed them 'The Respondents'.

I always feel on top of the world when babies are conceived in the bedroom rather than in the laboratory.

Take Home Message:

It is a lamentable and unfortunate fact that, since the advent of assisted reproductive technologies (ART) and IVF–ICSI, male factor evaluation often gets left out at many infertility centres. It is only the semen sample that gets examined, not the man. Since the male factor accounts for fifty per cent of all infertility, this is a major omission, as many causes of male infertility are curable. Couples seeking infertility treatment must insist on an andrological evaluation of the male partner.

27

The Umpteenth Time

When it comes to sex, aphorisms like 'the grass is always greener on the other side of the fence' and 'keeping up with the Joneses' are especially pertinent. Socially, it is quite common for close friends and relatives to exchange notes about their sex lives. Per se, there is nothing wrong with this practice. In fact, it constitutes an unofficial channel for sex education, offers opportunities for widening of one's sexual horizons, and can even provide some free entertainment. Besides, if something is drastically wrong with your own sex life, and you are not even aware of it because of ignorance and lack of previous experience, such gossip fora can be useful eye openers that prompt you to seek professional help.

There is, however, a flip side to this. People are notorious liars when it comes to talking about their sex lives, and will tell grossly exaggerated tales of their sexual prowess. The obvious aim of this braggadocio is to score one-upmanship points. The gullible listener usually falls for these tall tales hook, line and sinker, and starts to actually believe them. Since such conversations usually occur only among very close people, the trust quotient is high. The listener believes that if the teller is trusting him* with something so personal and intimate, he* must be definitely telling the truth. After all, who would expect a sister or best friend to lie about such personal matters? There is no apparent motive to do so. The listener also believes, therefore, that he must prove himself to be worthy of that trust and must never leak it out. And this is how these blatant sexual lies remain closely kept secrets. You can never cross check them. You remain forever in their grip.

You'll be surprised to know that this happens much more frequently than you might imagine. Thus, the people who are closest to you end up inflicting the maximum damage, albeit inadvertently.

If a guy tells you that his is ten inches long, or that he does it twelve times a night, or that his wife is so multi-orgasmic that she keeps twitching, writhing and convulsing all night long, chances are that you'll believe him and develop the complex of your life. You are never going to ask the guy to show you his penis, you are not going to peep into his bedroom, and you are not going to check with the wife whether the husband's description of her sexuality was accurate.

Thus, the guy laughs all the way back to his bedroom, smug in the knowledge that he has blown your mind out completely.

---

*Implies both genders

Let me tell you the story of this guy who once came to my clinic and said, 'Doc, I have a major problem when I try to do it the fourth time.'

I've heard worse. I didn't bat an eyelid. Instead, I looked him straight in the eye and asked him to elaborate on his story and tell more details. That was all the encouragement he needed. His verbal diarrhea lasted several minutes thereafter. Here's a summary:

'The first three times doc,' he began, 'I am somehow able to manage to get it up but the fourth time around, it is well nigh impossible. My wife is very co-operative and tries hard to stimulate me but still I can't do it.'

The word 'co-operative' is one that I hear very commonly in my consulting room. It seems to be particularly characteristic of Indian women who sleep with sexually inept men. In short, it means that the woman puts up with lousy sexual performances and sexual dissatisfaction, night after night, year after year, without any complaints. To 'co-operate' apparently also means 'to observe silently and say encouraging things as the man makes a complete fool of himself in bed'. Believe me, there are millions of 'co-operative' Indian women out there. I have often wondered why they've never started a 'Non-co-operation' movement like our freedom fighters did.

So then I asked our Charlie why it was so important for him to do it a fourth time. Weren't his wife and he happy with three times?

'Not at all, doc,' he said gloomily. 'You see, the very first time around, I ejaculate even before I enter. The second time, I ejaculate as soon as I enter. Even the third time, I'm not much better and last only two or three strokes. My wife is extremely dissatisfied and often hasn't even begun to get aroused.'

That was very easy for me to understand. But what I will never understand is how such wives are still very 'co-operative'! Are they not aware of their right to sexual fulfilment? Can't they tell their partners what they'd like in bed? Can't they speak up for their needs? Why must they pretend that everything is all right when it isn't? Are they embarrassed to admit that they want to enjoy sex? Do they think enjoying good sex is amoral? Do they think that their partners will consider them less virtuous if they are vocal, experimental, and demanding about sex?

'For God's sake!' I feel like telling them, 'Even the World Health Organization (WHO) has declared sexual health a fundamental health right. Why are you people still living in the Dark Ages? Don't you watch *The Bold and the Beautiful*? Haven't you seen all those brazenly sexual babes flaunting it in the music remix channels? When are you going to address, discover, and sate your sexual urges?'

Charlie went on to say that his wife's friend had once told her that the friend's husband could do it seven to eight times a night. 'And I can't even do it four times,' he concluded woefully. I didn't have the heart to tell him that, as per my understanding, he does not do it properly even once. That would have finished him completely.

Instead, I told him that he need not worry so much and that his problem was an eminently curable one. I told him that he was making a mistake trying to engage in the numbers' game. It was not how many times one did it that mattered but how well.

I said that if he did it properly even once such that both his wife and he were satisfied, it would be more than enough. I explained to him what foreplay is, what a woman's erogenous zones are, and taught him a thing or two about breast and clitoris stimulation. I also told him that he was very lucky to have a 'co-operative' wife. I did not tell him that her co-operation might not last too long if he didn't get his act together in a hurry. He was in a bad way already. No point making it worse. 'That's not what he's come to me for,' I thought to myself.

I then went on to further explain to him that his most important problem was premature ejaculation and that we should first work towards resolving that. I taught him all the techniques and exercises that are described in *On Fast Guys and other Seminal Matters*. I wrote him a prescription for medicines that would improve both erection and ejaculation. The consultation lasted nearly half an hour. At the end of it, he nodded with relief and hope as he left my office confidently.

A few weeks later, his plight had improved considerably and he was able to have a fairly normal sex life. His wife, who accompanied him this time, endorsed this and said that she was not just being 'co-operative', but that she was really happy now. Apparently, Charlie had worked hard, both on himself and on her (pun intended).

It is important for couples to understand that they should work at a sex life that works for them and not try to emulate others. Every relationship is different.

So, do you still have a 'co-operative' wife? If you do, then please call my secretary immediately for an appointment.

28

The Sex Addict

Recently, a visibly tormented gentleman came to see me. He began without much prelude.

'You see, doctor, I am a married man with a great wife and two lovely children but I just can't stop having affairs. I seem to be obsessed with sex. Over the past few years, I have had several illicit liaisons and I'm just going from one woman to another. Right now, I'm in four parallel relationships. Yet, I feel dissatisfied, empty and filled with remorse and guilt. I'm just not able to stop. I am exhausted and I need help. I don't want to break my family or ruin any more relationships. I know the dangers of promiscuity but yet seem to lose all reason and self-control when it matters most. I'm tired of leading a life full of duplicity and deceit. Even my work has now started suffering.'

Mr Satyromaniac's was a classical textbook case. 'Hmm...' I said, 'At least you've admitted your problem to yourself and sought professional help. That's half the battle won,' I said reassuringly. Whereupon, I reached into my drawer and pulled out the Sex

Addicts Anonymous' twelve-point sexual addiction self-test quiz. A 'Yes' to more than one of the twelve questions was advised professional help. Mr Satyromaniac said 'Yes' to seven!

Sex addiction is an increasingly recognised social problem. Nearly eight per cent of men and three per cent of women suffer sexual addiction. In the USA alone, there are an estimated fifteen million sex addicts! The list includes celebrities like Michael Douglas (now cured).

What exactly is sex addiction?

The brain's perception of and response to pain and stress (and their relief) is to a large extent controlled by substances within, known as endorphins and encephalins. These substances relieve pain and promote a feeling of well-being. Addictive drugs act by releasing these same chemicals in the brain. Sex is one of the most potent triggers for the release of endorphins and encephalins. Hence the human propensity for sexual addiction. Put to good use, sex is enriching. If abused, it can be destructive, like any other contraband substance. The sex addict has learnt to rely on sex for comfort from pain, for nurturing, or relief from stress — much like the alcoholic's purposeful use of alcohol — rather than enjoying sex as a self-affirming source of physical pleasure.

The essence of all addiction is the addicts' sense of powerlessness over a compulsive behaviour, resulting in the addicts' lives becoming unmanageable. The addict is out of control and experiences tremendous shame, pain and self-loathing. The addict may wish to stop, yet, repeatedly fails to do so. The unmanageability of the addicts' lives can be seen in the consequences they suffer — losing relationships, difficulties with work, arrests, financial troubles, a loss of interest in things not sexual, low self-esteem and despair. Common manifestations of sexual addiction include compulsive masturbation, obsession with sexual fantasy and/ or pornography, sex with prostitutes, anonymous sex with multiple partners, multiple affairs, frequent patronising of topless bars or sexual massage parlours, exhibitionism, voyeurism, inappropriate sexual touching including frotteurism, sexual abuse of children and rape.

The beginnings of sexual addiction are usually rooted in adolescence or childhood. The child often grows up in a chaotic, hostile or neglectful home and turns repeatedly to masturbation to escape this environment. Masturbation becomes a regular sedative for the child. Alternatively, the child may be introduced to sex in inappropriate ways — by an adult, older cousin, baby-sitter, etc., where the sexual experience does not feel mutual. In such situations, there is a combination of natural curiosity, new-found pleasurable feelings and also feelings of fear and shame. When the child grows up, he/she may be turned on by sex in high-risk situations that unconsciously generate fear, or in secretive circumstances that feed on shame. Recent research has shown that nearly sixty per cent of adult sex addicts were sexually abused by someone during their childhood.

Though challenging, the condition is curable, like any other drug addiction. Help is also available on the internet and through support groups.

As for Mr Satyromaniac, he has now mended his ways considerably and is on the path to recovery.

29

Sad in the Sack

Recently, a young couple came to see me. The man's face seemed oddly familiar. Where had I seen him...? And then, in a flash, I got it. SAD SACK! Yes, that's who he was. I have read just too many of Sad Sack's comics in my childhood to make a wrong diagnosis. It was truly unbelievable. This man looked like he was going to burst into tears any minute.

'It's obvious that something's wrong,' I began insightfully, 'What is it?'

'What *isn't* wrong might be a more appropriate question, doctor,' said the wife, spewing fire. She looked like an angry volcano on the verge of an eruption. I told myself that I'd better tread carefully. This was land mine territory.

'It's been two years since we got married, but I'm still a virgin,' she said.

'Aah, that explains it!' I thought to myself, not one bit surprised. 'And why is that so?' I asked.

It turned out that Mr Sad Sack had been suffering from depression for the past several years. He was brilliant at his job, albeit highly stressed. He had been put on high doses of anti-depressant medication — a combination of fluoxetine and sertraline (both SSRI or Selective Serotonin Reuptake Inhibitor drugs). He now had no libido or desire whatsoever, no erections, and couldn't even ejaculate. Hardly surprising, therefore, that Ms Volcano was still a virgin. It took four months to solve Mr Sad Sack's problem. He was advised to go for counselling and his anti-depressant medication doses were gradually tapered until he was finally weaned off them. With a little help from other oral medication and penile injections, the marriage was finally consummated.

Depression is, according to many experts, the most common, under-diagnosed and under-treated disease among humans. It can cause sexual dysfunction in both sexes. Mild depression in men is associated with a 42.3 per cent incidence of overall impotence and the figure goes up to 100 per cent for major depression. The additional bad news is that many drugs used to treat depression themselves can affect libido and orgasm adversely, thus compounding the problem. Recently, depression has also been shown to co-exist with cardiovascular disease and erectile dysfunction in the form of a clinical triad, or a disease entity where all three conditions occur together in the same patient.

SSRIs have revolutionised the treatment of depression during the past few years. This class of antidepressants includes such drugs as Prozac® (fluoxetine), Paxil® (paroxetine), and

Zoloft® (sertraline). In India, these same drugs are marketed under several different generic names. But even when SSRIs are prescribed to appropriate patients, they are not perfect. Recently, researchers have found that adverse sexual side effects, notably libido loss and orgasmic difficulty, can occur in fifty per cent of those taking SSRIs. So, if you're on an SSRI and you're suddenly having sexual problems, the medicine might be to blame. And it's time to talk to your doctor about it.

Many physicians fail to mention the potential sexual side effects of SSRIs to their patients. Perhaps this is because they are not aware of recent studies, don't want to scare patients, or are simply short on time. Without being warned about the side effects, patients may have no idea that their problems could be related to the medicines.

However, there are solutions. Stopping the medicine usually solves the sexual problem, but for safety this should only be done under a doctor's supervision. A physician who suspects SSRI-related sexual dysfunction may also consider lowering the dose, switching to a non-SSRI anti-depressant, or suggesting that the patient take a drug holiday. For instance, a patient who hopes to have sex on Saturday evening might stop taking the drug a few days before, depending on how long the specific drug stays in the bloodstream.

How well these strategies work depends on the specific drug and the individual patient. Complicating the doctor's decision about what to do is the possibility that the depression itself might be causing the sexual problems. In addition, there is lack of agreement and knowledge among doctors about how to best treat

SSRI-related sexual dysfunction, because the problem is newly recognised.

But the bottom line, for anyone on an SSRI, is that no one should sacrifice sexual satisfaction for psychological health without first exploring what can be done. Hopefully, you can have both a good sex life and psychological well-being.

Meantime, I'm told that Ms Volcano still erupts, but for entirely different reasons nowadays.

30

The Suffering Companion

Some days ago, a heavily made-up forty-something lady came to see me at my office. Trailing her like miasma was a pungent floral fragrance. I winced.

'Am I not attractive...?' she started abruptly.

I started too.

I always seem to find myself in such difficult situations. If I said I thought she was indeed attractive, it might have been misconstrued. If I told her she wasn't, that would've been certain catastrophe too, considering how formidable she looked.

'How is that andrologically pertinent?' I asked instead, trying to embody professionalism at its best.

'No, no doc, my husband thinks that I am not attractive and to think I was a beauty contest winner in college...it really hurts ' She broke into sobs.

'I'm sorry ma'am, but I'm not a cosmetic surgeon', I had to finally confess.

'No, no, you don't seem to understand, doc,' she persisted and pulled out some sheets of paper from her commodious purse. 'The case histories you describe here are exactly like ours — my husband's and mine, that is.'

I took the papers from her and perused them. They were printouts from the chapter on my website on the woman's perspective of impotence.

'I see,' I muttered. This was getting interesting.

'My husband and I have been married twenty-eight years', she said, 'but for the past two years, there has been no sex whatsoever. He never initiates sex nowadays. Even if I try, he just doesn't respond in spite of all my caresses and stimulation. He says he's sorry but he can't do it and that it doesn't matter if we can't have sex. But I know that it does matter. And so does he.'

Any woman who has tried to have intercourse with an impotent man can identify with Ms Sexless' feelings. It isn't just men who experience frustration and disappointment. Women do too.

Many couples maintain a conspiracy of silence surrounding the problem of impotence. Mr and Ms Sexless both knew there was a problem, but typically were reluctant to talk about it. Neither man nor wife was willing to accept the reality of impotence. They were caught in a double bind. If they openly addressed the issue, much anxiety and stress would be generated. If they chose to ignore the problem, opportunities for emotional and sexual closeness would be lost. As they became more physically distant, the quality of their marital relationship began to deteriorate. Over time, they gradually began to drift apart. Silence reinforced their estrangement.

The story of Mr and Ms Sexless is classical. Millions of couples languish in silent misery or endure deteriorating marriages when the husband is impotent. But this need not be so because the situation is eminently remediable. Here's a six-step survival guide:

Step 1: Examine the Effects of Impotence on You and Your Relationship:

This includes, first, admitting the problem to yourselves and then examining your feelings, your thoughts and beliefs, and your behaviour. Are you blaming yourself and your lack of attractiveness for your husband's problem? Are you suspecting your husband to be having an affair? Are you ignoring, denying or making excuses for the problem? Are you withholding affection and avoiding sexual situations? Are you seeking escapism through over-exercising, overeating, alcohol or spiritual pursuits?

None of these will help solve your problem.

Step 2: Consider your Physical and Psychological Health:

Determine what kind of sexuality is appropriate for your age and act accordingly. Are there any underlying diseases that need treatment? Is medication/depression interfering with your sex life?

Step 3: Explore the Relationship Factors that Predict Successful Treatment:

The most important issue here is: 'Are you committed to working with your partner on solving this problem? Is your partner motivated to work with you?' This is crucial.

Step 4: Learn about the Causes and Treatment Options for Impotence:

Impotence has many physical causes and several treatment options. Educate yourself about them.

Step 5: Discuss the Problem with your Mate and Seek Medical Consultation:

The sooner you do this, the better.

Step 6: See an Andrologist:

Get an expert to identify the cause of your partner's erectile dysfunction and offer case-specific treatment. Sometimes, surgery may be necessary.

31

Paraphilias

Paraphilias are problems with controlling impulses that are characterised by recurrent and intense sexual fantasies, urges, and behaviours involving unusual objects, activities, or situations not considered sexually arousing to others. The individual's urges and behaviours cause significant distress and/or personal, social or occupational dysfunction. They may have serious social and legal consequences.

Exhibitionism

Exhibitionism is characterised by exposure of the individual's genitals to an unsuspecting stranger. The exhibitionist, sometimes called a 'flasher', feels a need to surprise, shock or impress his victims. The condition is usually limited to the exposure, with no other harmful advances made. Actual sexual contact with the victim is rare. However, the person may masturbate while exposing himself.

Fetishism

People with this problem have sexual urges associated with non-living objects. The person becomes sexually aroused by wearing or touching the object. For example, the object of a fetish could be women's shoes, women's underwear or lingerie.

Frotteurism

In frotteurism, the focus of the person's sexual urges is related to touching or rubbing his genitals against the body of a non-consenting, unfamiliar person. In most cases, a male rubs his genitals against a female, often in a crowded public location.

Paedophilia

People with this problem have behaviours that involve illegal sexual activity with prepubescent children. Paedophilic behaviour includes undressing the child, encouraging the child to watch the abuser masturbate, touching or fondling the child's genitals and forcefully performing sexual acts on the child. Some limit their activity to their own children or close relatives (incest), while others victimise other children. Predatory paedophiles may use force or threaten their victims if they disclose the abuse.

Masochism

Individuals with this disorder use sexual behaviours involving the act of being humiliated, beaten or otherwise made to suffer in order to achieve sexual excitement. These acts may be limited to verbal humiliation, or may involve being beaten, bound or otherwise abused. Masochists may act out their fantasies on themselves — such as cutting or piercing their skin, or burning themselves — or may seek out a partner who enjoys inflicting pain or humiliation on others (sadist). Activities with a partner include bondage, spanking, and simulated rape.

Sadism

Individuals with this disorder have persistent fantasies in which sexual excitement results from inflicting psychological or physical suffering (including humiliation and terror) on a sexual partner. In some cases, sexual sadists are able to find willing partners to participate in the sadistic activities. At its most extreme, sexual sadism involves illegal activities such as rape, torture and even murder, in which case the death of the victim produces sexual excitement. These individuals need intensive psychiatric treatment and may be jailed.

Transvestism

Transvestism refers to the practice by heterosexual persons of dressing in clothes traditionally associated with the opposite sex to produce or enhance sexual arousal. This usually does not involve a real partner, but includes the fantasy that the individual is the female partner, as well. Some men wear only one special piece of female clothing, such as underwear, while others fully dress as female, including hair-style and make-up. Cross-dressing itself is not a problem, unless it is necessary for the individual to become sexually aroused or experience sexual climax.

Voyeurism (Peeping Tom)

This disorder involves achieving sexual arousal by observing an unsuspecting and non-consenting person who is undressing or unclothed, and/or engaged in sexual activity. This behaviour may conclude with masturbation by the voyeur. The voyeur does not seek sexual contact with the person he is observing.

Urolagnia/Coprophilia

These are perversions where the person gets aroused by the sight or smell of, or contact with urine and stools, during sexual activity.

Paraphilias are uncommon, and are more prevalent among males than females (about twenty to one). It is not known for certain what causes paraphilia. Many paraphilias begin during adolescence and continue into adulthood. Most cases are treated with counselling and therapy. Medication may help to decrease the compulsiveness associated with paraphilia, and reduce the number of deviant sexual fantasies and behaviours. Treatment must be on a long-term basis. Unwillingness to comply with treatment can hinder its success. It is imperative that people with paraphilia of an illegal nature receive professional help before they harm others or create legal problems for themselves.

32

Sex during Pregnancy

I receive a lot of queries from pregnant ladies about the safety of having sex during pregnancy. I usually ask them to consult their obstetricians, of course, but for those who are shy, embarrassed or plain lazy, here's a ready reckoner of FAQs.

Can I have sex during pregnancy without harming my baby?

There is no reason to change your sexual activity during pregnancy unless your doctor advises otherwise. Intercourse or orgasm during pregnancy will not harm your baby, unless you have a medical problem. Remember that your baby is well protected in your uterus by the amniotic fluid that surrounds it.

Your doctor may recommend not having intercourse early in pregnancy if you have a history of miscarriages. Intercourse may also be restricted if you have certain complications of pregnancy, such as pre-term labour or bleeding. You may need to ask your doctor and clarify whether this means no penetration, no orgasms, or no sexual arousal, as different complications may require different restrictions.

How can I stay comfortable during intercourse?

As your pregnancy progresses, changing positions may become necessary for your comfort. This also may be true after your baby is born.

A water-based lubricant may be used during intercourse if necessary.

During intercourse, you should not feel pain. During orgasm, your uterus will contract. If you have any contractions that are painful or irregular, please contact your doctor. Also, discontinue intercourse and call your doctor immediately if you have heavy vaginal bleeding or if your water breaks. *Nothing*, not even your naughty husband's naughty penis, should enter the vagina after your water breaks.

Talking to your partner about how you are feeling about sex and any concerns you have will help you stay comfortable. Also, encourage your partner to communicate with you, especially if you notice changes in his responsiveness. Communicating can help you both better understand your feelings and desires.

Will my desires change?

It is common for your desires to be different now that you are pregnant. Changing hormones cause some women to experience an increased sex drive during pregnancy, while others may not be as interested in sex as they were before.

During the first trimester, some women commonly lose interest in sex because they are tired and uncomfortable (or puke-y), while other women's desires stay the same.

I don't feel like having sex. What should I do to keep my partner happy?

If your doctor has limited your sexual activity, or if you are not in the mood for intercourse, remember to spend other time with your partner. Being intimate does not always require having intercourse — love and affection can be expressed in many ways.

Remind yourselves of the love that created your developing baby. Enjoy your time together. You can take long romantic walks, enjoy candle-lit dinners or give each other back rubs.

How soon can I have sex after my baby is born?

In general, you can resume sexual activity when you have recovered, when your bleeding has stopped, and when you and your partner feel comfortable.

Your doctor may recommend that you wait until after your first post-partum doctor appointment before having intercourse with your partner.

After pregnancy, some women notice a lack of vaginal lubrication during intercourse. A water-based lubricant may be used.

Women who only feed their babies breast milk, experience a delay in ovulation (when an egg is released from the ovary) and menstruation. But ovulation will occur before you start having menstrual periods again, so remember that you can still become pregnant during this time. Follow your doctor's recommendation on the appropriate method of birth control to use.

And now, the secret and the real reason behind this article!

Basically, this piece is addressed to those all-too-eager husbands of pregnant women who have a one-track mind. You must try and understand that though sex during pregnancy can be safe and enjoyable at most times, there are plenty of situations where the lady can have anxieties, discomfort, or simply a lost libido. One must try to be considerate and adjusting. And how does one do that?

Simple. Try and take matters in your own hands. Sometimes it is necessary to spare the rod so as not to spoil the child!

33

Sex after a Heart Attack

Men who have experienced a heart attack are often concerned and anxious about having sex in the months and years following it. Research has shown that sexual activity often decreases because of the fear that it may cause another heart attack, possibly leading to death.

Men also report higher levels of erectile dysfunction (ED, impotence) and decreased levels of sexual contact than prior to the attack. A heart attack is a dramatic event in anyone's life and often comes as a complete shock. The changes such an event can have on the way you think and behave are often profound. In many cases, these changes are good and result in some positive life benefits. However, unfounded fears are counter-productive. So what should you do?

Be realistic. Seek out advice to any questions you have and get the information and advice from health care professionals so that you can lead a full and successful life following a heart attack. But do you have to talk about your sex life to someone you hardly know? Well, yes and no.

Following a heart attack, health professionals should know that you will want guidance on a number of issues and they should advise you on lifestyle, medications, exercise and sex. The topic of sex can be a difficult subject for both the patient and medical staff and the subject is often avoided. Yet, it is vital that you get the information so that you can make a complete recovery — so ask.

Does one need to worry?

Think of it this way. Sex, in general, puts the same amount of pressure on the heart as a brisk twenty-minute walk, and the orgasm adds up to a walk up the stairs. Statistics suggest that only one per cent of heart attacks are triggered by sexual activity. If you have had a heart attack and have made lifestyle changes that lead to a healthier you, then the odds should go even further in your favour! Do you stop going up the stairs or going for a brisk walk because you have a one per cent chance of another heart attack? No you do not.

Exercise is good for the heart and sexual activity is just another form of exercise. So, contrary to some men's fears, regular sexual activity actually protects against death, especially death resulting from heart attack.

How long should one wait before having sexual intercourse following a heart attack?

This will depend on the severity of the heart attack. Tests will have been done prior to your discharge from hospital as to the cause and extent of damage to the heart. A progressive structure of exercise and advice on any changes to diet, such as fat reduction, weight loss or low salt, quitting smoking, and a regime of medication, will also have been advised. The only way to find out specifics from your doctor is by asking questions. This is especially true about sex. Most doctors will say that as long as no adverse symptoms such as breathlessness or chest pains are experienced on exertion (climbing stairs, a brisk walk), resuming sexual activity will be safe.

What if I do get chest pains or breathlessness?

If you do find that you get chest pains (angina) or breathlessness, then you should discuss it with your doctor. He/she may suggest you take medication such as sublingual glyceryl trinitrate. It could, of course, also be that your anxiety and fear are causing the symptoms and if this is the case then supportive advice should alleviate your worries. If you still experience problems then the doctor should refer you for more specialist help.

If you are suffering from co-existent erectile dysfunction (ED), you will need to see your andrologist. He might want to medicate you with one or more of the newly available wonder drugs like Viagra®*, Levitra®, or Cialis® for your ED. Please remember, however, that if you are on nitrates for your heart disease, it can be dangerous to take these drugs*. With good medical follow up and support there should be no reason why you should not return to a full sex life.

Two closing thoughts

Cardiologist Dr Graham Jackson has found that seventy-five per cent of deaths that do occur during sexual intercourse are in people having extramarital affairs and in men who are much older than their sexual partners!

So watch out, you naughty boys! It seems that you might have to choose where you want all your blood to go — to your heart, or 'that part'.

Take Home Message:

Shortly after the launch of Viagra® in March 1998, there was some unfounded initial concern about its safety in some patient populations, especially in those with co-existent heart disease. Some adverse reports began to appear in the media about side-effects and deaths in some patients who had taken Viagra®. A fear psychosis of sorts was generated. Soon, however, the US FDA stepped in, and the American Heart Association (AHA), the American Urological Association (AUA), and the American College of Cardiology (ACC) were called in to investigate these 'side effects' and 'deaths'. The investigation revealed that most of these adverse reactions were caused not by the drug per se at all, but by careless patients and doctors who did not follow the prescription guidelines, safety precautions, and warning labels. Those taking nitrates and others who were not supposed to be taking Viagra® at all in the first place had taken it, doses had been exceeded without medical advice, and some prescriptions had been issued by unscrupulous practitioners through the internet without even examining the patient's medical history.

The current position on this subject is available in the Princeton Consensus Conference Statements (Guidelines) I and II. The safety/ risk aspects of the relationship between heart disease, sex and the new PDE5 inhibitor drugs are discussed in great detail.

It is now known that many cardiac patients with heart disease and erectile dysfunction can use these new drugs safely to obtain better erections and enjoy a satisfactory sex life.

Patients and doctors should both learn to feel more comfortable discussing this subject.

34

Gain One Organ, Lose Another

One of the fringe benefits of medical practice is that one gets to meet a lot of new and interesting people in the course of work. Otherwise, practice itself can get quite monotonous, especially if one has chosen to restrict oneself to a small sub-specialty such as mine, where data are often quite repetitive. I try and make the best of these interaction opportunities to break the tedium and learn new things.

Some days ago, a man walked in with his young (late teens/early twenties) daughter. They made an odd couple. The man looked like a typical prosperous Indian businessman. He was dressed in a shiny white safari suit with the top button open to reveal a hairy chest, wore white slippers and silver spectacles, sported a flashy watch, and was bejewelled with gold rings and chains. He also incessantly chewed *Pan Parag* or equivalent and spoke only in the vernacular. As a bumper bonus, he provided additional special effects with a continuous oscillation of a leg and one white leather slipper tapping on the floor metronomically.

By contrast, his daughter was a picture of calm dignity and composure. She was smartly dressed and looked educated. It was she, I believe, who wanted to meet me. She seemed very keen to start talking and didn't wait for an invitation.

'Good evening doc, I have come here to obtain some clarifications,' she began. 'My parents are talking of getting me married to a man who is the son of old family friends of ours. We are childhood pals and it was taken for granted by all that we would marry when we grew up. They are planning the engagement in a few months.'

'That certainly sounds very romantic, like an Indian film,' I said, wrongly supposing that she had come to me for some pre-marital sex education and contraception or fertility advice, like many do.

'It only *sounds* romantic, doctor,' she shot back sharply, 'I'm afraid that if I don't take the right steps in a timely manner, it might end up being everything *but* that.'

Nothing flippant about this kid. Youngsters these days are so focussed. It was not like this in my time. We were totally clueless about life at her age. All these thoughts were passing through my mind. The girl shook me out of my reverie by speaking again.

'You see, doctor, my prospective fiancé has undergone a kidney transplant about a year ago. The operation has gone off quite well and, for all practical purposes, he's more or less back to a normal life, but I'm given to understand that after a renal transplant some of the important practical purposes of marriage cannot be fulfilled. Am I right?'

I liked both her curious brand of modesty and her strange syntax and wanted to ask whether she had majored in English but circumstances just didn't seem propitious. Can't be facetious when a patient is dead serious, I told myself. It sends all the wrong signals. I turned to concentrate on the situation before me.

'Yes, you are right,' I told her, 'According to some experts, as many as eighty-seven per cent of patients are impotent after a renal transplant operation. But how did you know this? This is not well-known, even among doctors. In fact, most doctors are notorious for not even addressing the sex lives of their renal failure patients. On the other hand, we andrologists think only of that and nothing else. What a contrast!'

'Doctor, I remember you had mentioned in one of your earlier columns that kidney failure can cause impotence. After reading that, I read some more books and even surfed the internet. It became some kind of an obsession. After all, this was an extremely important decision for me. I discussed it with my parents and showed them some informative material, but they wouldn't hear of it. Finally, I asked dad to come along with me to meet you. Please explain to him, will you?'

I then told Mr Metronome that chronic renal failure (CRF) is one of the commonest causes of impotence and that it can also cause libido impairment, ejaculatory disturbances, decreased penile sensation and low sperm counts. Almost every component of the sexual apparatus is affected — small arteries, large arteries, veins, penile smooth muscle, nerves and hormones. The problem is further compounded by the co-existence of diabetes, hypertension and depression along with CRF and the many drugs that are used to treat all these conditions. Transplantation restores hormonal levels, libido, ejaculatory function and sperm counts in many. However, many continue to remain impotent. Generally, there is very little awareness about this co-existence. So, many men gain one organ, but lose another.

Right now, Mr Fiancé (whom Mr Metronome kept referring to as 'Fancy') is awaiting a penile prosthetic implantation operation and is hoping that, for all practical purposes, he can fulfil all practical purposes within marriage soon after surgery.

I was very optimistic that the young lady would finally be happy. She had worked hard to achieve it, and deserved every bit of it.

Take Home Message:

When people are battling serious illnesses, we doctors (and relatives) often forget that behind the patient there is a person and a sexual being. Often, there is also a partner involved. However, the serious nature of the immediate illness is such that it pushes any consideration of sex completely out of the picture.

However, with modern treatment methods, many serious illnesses are considerably curable, and when these patients return to some semblance of a normal life after treatment, sex again becomes an important need. Often, people do not even connect that the illness itself has worsened the sex life. They simply think that the patient has lost interest in sex. But mostly, they don't think about sex at all! Thus, this need is either never addressed or, even if it is, the sexual problem is thought to be incurable.

It is important to recognise that patients with illnesses are also sexual beings and that their sexual requirements need to be addressed. It is even more important to recognise that most patients are treatable and can resume nearly normal sex lives after treatment.

35

Where has Desire Gone?

Sex. The passion, intimacy, fun, games, naughtiness — could you live without it? Yet, everywhere, couples are doing without sex because, frankly, they're not in the mood. What was once a wonderful three times a night has dwindled to a routine once a week, half-hearted once a month or even less. Here are the reasons why one might go off sex.

Your physical self

Firstly, are you feeling good physically? We may lust with our minds but it's our bodies that have to do the lovemaking. So if you're tired, stressed, overworked or ill, you may not feel like sex simply because your body isn't up to it. Begin by making sure you're getting enough rest. Work, stress, a house to keep and children often lead to feelings of exhaustion. If you have children, try going to bed when they do for a week. Or clear your diary for a week to ensure early nights. Catch up on sleep and see how much better you feel. Lack of desire may be your body's way of telling you there's something wrong. It could be illness that's draining you or your hormones may be unbalanced. Or you're on medication that's reducing your sex drive. It's always worth having a physical check-up, particularly if your problems have come on suddenly after many years of normal sex. In such situations, the cause is more likely to be physical than psychological.

Relationship frustration

Falling in love and having lots of sex go hand in hand. If your love starts to dip, often you won't long for as much sex. So, while it may feel strange to question your relationship, you do need to look at it. Do you still have a working partnership? Are you still in love? If in your heart you know you're not, be brave enough to admit it to yourself. Even if you know you do still love and care, you might be suffering from the biggest enemy of desire — anger. Over the years, many things may have happened to make you irritated with each other. From the betrayal of an affair to a series of small irritations, disagreements, rows, perhaps a whole range of disappointments — and neither partner feels loved or wanted. This build up of anger will block all sexual feeling, and so desire dies. The only solution is to dissolve this anger, which is not necessarily an easy process. You need to identify what you are angry about — and the list may be long. Ideally, talk these issues through with your partner, clear the air, forgive each other and then learn ways to stop anger building up again. If you can't discuss issues with your partner without tempers exploding, then a counsellor can help you. Of course, sexual frequency and intensity also decline in long-standing relationships as people age. This is normal and you mustn't worry about it if the sex is acceptable to both partners.

Sexual reasons

Finally, your sex life may have faded because you're not enjoying it anymore. If you aren't having fun during sex, why bother having it? And if there are other things that are more fun than sex, then why bother having sex? We're not talking here about improving sex by using different positions, buying sex aids or dressing up in saucy knickers. These things will add spice to a good but routine sex life, but they won't bring desire back. The sexual reasons for loss of desire are far deeper. To begin with, it could be that you're no longer really turning each other on. Although men often like the 'straight in, no messing approach', for true pleasure, they need arousing. The best way is to go back to square one and 're-teach' each other turn-on skills. Do you need lots of foreplay, a gentle touch or stimulation in a certain way or a particular spot? Take it in turns to simply 'receive' touch — coaching your partner in what really works for you. Another problem, especially for women, may be inability to have orgasms — at least with the partner. This is very common. Many — if not most — women attain orgasm more easily alone than with a partner. This often happens because foreplay declines dramatically in a relationship with the passage of time. In such a situation, the woman can teach her partner how to bring her to climax.

So many men and women have lost interest in sex completely and are not even bothered about it. Yet, they've read every word of this piece!

Theory yes, practicals no, perhaps?

36

Passage to Manhood

Take a young girl of today and you'll be amazed at how much she knows about basic female sexuality. We're not talking about love-making skills and coital positions here, but about elementary reproductive biology. The ten or eleven-year-old girl knows about the bodily changes that are going to occur in her. She knows about menstruation, about how it is a cyclical, quintessentially feminine phenomenon, and about its sexual and reproductive implications. She knows what sex is, what sexual abuse is, how pregnancies and venereal diseases occur and about what precautions she must take as she grows up. This empiric knowledge exists even among girls from the most conservative homes.

By contrast, boys, even in the most educated, broad-minded and affluent families, are usually told very little in the name of sex education. 'Boys will learn on their own' seems to be the standard refrain. The irony here is that girls, thought to be the weaker sex that can be sexually exploited, are protectively taught about sexual matters in a timely manner.

Addressing sex itself, therefore, is perceived as a very sissy thing, only for girls, definitely not what one would want to do for one's macho son. Nobody taught the boys' fathers either, you see. The reality, of course, is that many fathers are extremely embarrassed about discussing sex with their boys. It would be also wrong to presume that the fathers know too much beyond mere peno-vaginal penetration. The poor boys, therefore, are left to fend for themselves.

Some 'progressive' fathers might tell their sons not to 'knock up' some girl and get into trouble. That's the only brand of sex education they know. Having said that, they'll guffaw, raise their glasses, and say 'cheers' to their friends seated around them. In some such extremely 'hep' environs, the boy, who is now a 'man', is offered his first drink, amidst much fanfare. This is considered an important rite of passage to manhood, never mind that the boy doesn't even know how children are born and can't understand what that sticky fluid is. This drinking part, you see, is damn important!

Some other unfortunate chappies have their mothers (grandmothers, even) telling them not to 'waste' semen and about how such wastage can cause serious weakness. Some are even told that semen is so precious that one drop of this vital fluid equals forty drops of blood. And that's a conservative estimate. Sometimes, one drop can equal several hundred millilitres. It all depends on the story-telling skills of the educator. Small wonder then, that guys get totally panicked every time they ejaculate. And if you consider the biological fact that a teenaged boy ejaculates rather frequently, you'll understand that there is a multitude of panicking kids out there, including some who genuinely imagine that they have one foot in the grave because they have lost 'too much' semen already, at such a young age!

Much of the (mis)information boys glean is from misinformed parents *(vide supra)*, relatives, friends, and pornographic material. The rest of the education is obtained on the streets, by trial and error, as they go along. It's therefore surprising that many men still manage to reach adult life in one piece and cope well sexually. What is not surprising at all, however, is how so many others lose their way and are warped — sexually, emotionally, mentally, and sometimes even physically.

Take a look at these case studies and you'll understand why and how.

TA, a light-eyed, fair boy, studied in a residential boys' school, where he lived in a dormitory. He was slightly younger than most of his peers and also a little slower in the attainment of secondary sexual characteristics, i.e. masculine voice, body hair, height, muscular development, etc. At thirteen, his seniors caught him and forcibly sodomised him. This became a ritual until he left school at fifteen. He could neither tell his parents nor his school authorities. Perhaps as a consequence of this, he had major problems adjusting himself in a heterosexual relationship later in life. He is still coping.

PSS, just sixteen, was taken out by older friends for an evening of drinking and frolic. All he could recall the next day was entering a sleazy bar. After that, he didn't remember anything. He awoke the next morning to find himself on a filthy cot in a brothel. He was so sloshed that the brothel servant boy had to accompany him home in a taxi. Unable to confide the whole truth in his parents, he sobbed uncontrollably for two full days. Soon after, he developed full-blown gonorrhoea and had to furtively seek treatment from a faraway GP, with stolen money. From my interviews with him, I am convinced that a part of him will forever remain misogynistic, maybe even misanthropic.

In many feudal cultures (and India abounds in these), indoctrination into manhood is through serial womanising. This is sometimes done in groups, where many boys share one commercial sex worker. Wanton sex is considered a true sign of manhood amongst such people, and women are merely sex objects. The latter is reflected in every aspect of their society, and includes their mothers and wives-to-be. Such guys also, by right, expect to be permitted several partners and mistresses after marriage. In return, of course, they expect monomaniacal monogamy from their wives. Such is the brand of sex education that these guys receive.

Until recently, it was possible, much of the time, to get away with indifference to, and inappropriateness in, male sex education. Times have changed and the apathy of yesteryears is not longer tolerated by future generations. It's best, therefore, to start sex education early in life, in an age appropriate manner. And sex education is not just about the birds and the bees, about basic reproductive biology or reproductive diseases. Sex is much more than that. It's about values, relationships, needs, duties, and even performance. In a fluid, new world, with its ever-changing social and gender dynamics, the importance of keeping up to date with such education cannot be over-emphasised.

Of course, it must be reiterated that sexuality is just one aspect of growing up. As a man, you will, hopefully, have a lot more to do than just sex. But I can't help you with those responsibilities. Ask your mom and dad!

37

Horny, Healthy Oldies

Anti-ageing creams and plastic surgery aren't necessarily the best answers to staying young and healthy. The key, it seems, is sex — and lots of it. Recent research reveals that sex is the secret ingredient for successful ageing. A Sheffield University study on sexual relationships and sexual health among older people suggests that not only does sex get better with age, but older people who are having sex regularly have better physical and mental health than their chaste counterparts.

This revelation probably comes as a surprise to many people, particularly in India, where sex is traditionally considered the province of the young. Sex in your thirties, forties or even fifties is okay. But sex when you are over sixty? Unthinkable! Many of us have grown up with the idea that anyone over sixty who still has sex must be a dirty old man or woman. Crinkly sex is at best unseemly, and at worst downright repulsive. Our aversion to the idea that older people might enjoy and need sex is linked to our preconceived notions. It has to do with the stereotypes that we have about older people, namely, that they are asexual. This subject hasn't been researched in the past because of the erroneous assumption that older people would be unwilling and embarrassed to talk about sex. Hence, the whole subject was considered taboo and out of bounds. However, it has been shown that older people are actually very much prepared to talk about their feelings, and in fact, are often delighted to do so. It is just that no one had ever expressed an interest in this aspect of their lives before.

The Sheffield study shows that the Joan Collins Syndrome (the phenomenon of women who stay sexually active in their later years) is alive and well. It was clearly shown in the study that women, more than men, found that sex remained important to them as they aged. Older women have gone through the menopause and don't have to worry about contraception any more. They think about sex as something for enjoyment rather than something that is intimately connected with procreation, and this is very liberating for them. They might look at themselves and see that they are a bit saggy or wrinkly, but the fact that they still feel wanted by someone else makes them feel better about themselves. Besides, except in *The Bold and the Beautiful*, their partners are usually in the same age group too, and are as saggy and wrinkly. That makes it easier for both parties.

There is additional evidence to suggest that having sex when you are older can actually prolong your life. In 1997, a study published in the *British Medical Journal* examined the relationship between frequency of orgasm and mortality. It found that mortality was fifty per cent lower in the group with higher orgasmic occurrence than in the group with lower orgasmic frequency. Simply put, this suggests that the more orgasms you have, the longer you are likely to live. It is clear that sex and health appear to reinforce each other.

Due to advances in medical knowledge and a greater understanding of preventive health, we are all living longer and leading more active lives. Older people may not want to do it sixty-nine ways on a water bed, but neither do they want to be left on the bed, waiting until their time is up. Figures published in the Archives of Sexual Behaviour revealed that among healthy eighty to 102-year-olds, sixty-three per cent of men and thirty per cent of women are still having sexual intercourse. In this age group there are thirty-nine men for every 100 women, which may explain the difference. It doesn't mean that our ladies are any less horny! It thus appears that a few extra years on your clock doesn't make you any less of a person or a sexual being.

At the time of writing, we do not yet have proper published studies and figures about geriatric sexuality in India, though they are on their way already. But no matter what these studies might eventually show, and what the attitudinal and other differences between the Indian oldie and his/her western counterpart might be, it would be wrong to assume that all our senior citizens are abstemious ascetics. My oldest patient till date is an eighty-six-year-old man who had just married a much younger woman many years after the death of his first wife.

Geriatric sexuality is real, and must be respected and addressed.

So, guys, the scientific evidence seems to suggest that the best way to delay going (to heaven or hell) is by coming!

Take Home Message:

Ageing, geriatric sexuality, and gender matters are the theme subjects of India's new medical society, AGASSI. AGASSI stands for the Ageing, Gender, Andrology and Sexual (Sciences) Society of India. The interested reader is referred to *http://www.agassi.in* for further information about the association, its aims and objectives, memberships, and forthcoming conferences.

38

The Better Orgasm Diet

These days, everyone talks about natural remedies and positive health, i.e. that good health is not merely the absence of disease or infirmity. Allopathic medicines seem to be *passé*. So, for now, I've decided to switch bandwagons, give you a break from morbid medical terminology and cures, and take a peek at some 'natural' and 'positive' sexual cures.

Here goes...

If you want hotter sex, 'bypass the bedroom and head straight for the kitchen' is the new mantra. What you eat (or don't eat) has a direct impact on your sex life, affecting your hormone, energy and stress levels. Here are seven expert-certified foods to eat on your way to an explosive love life. This kind of explosion, I believe, has not yet been banned by governments.

1. **Honey:** The sweet stuff is a bountiful source of boron (a mineral also found in green leafy vegetables, fruits, legumes and nuts). Boron helps the body metabolise and utilise oestrogen,

the basic female sex hormone. Some studies have shown that this mineral may also enhance blood levels of testosterone, the hormone responsible for promoting the specific drive for genital sex and orgasm in both men and women.

2. **Walnut Oil:** Fats from vegetables, seeds, and nuts are key sources of fatty acids, from which your body produces cholesterol. Despite its bad reputation, cholesterol is the basis for all sex hormones. If you have recently started a rigorous non-fat diet and you've noticed a flagging of interest and desire, fit in more healthy fats and you'll probably experience a jump in libido. Look for vegetable and nut oils labelled 'cold-pressed'. These retain more nutrients than those processed with heat. Cold-pressed oils also contain vitamin E, which is essential to keeping your hormones balanced.

3. **Oats:** This equine favourite increases the amount of the hormone testosterone available in the blood. To pump up your libido, herbalists recommend eating a cup of cooked oatmeal and drinking three cups of oat-straw infusion a few times a week. To make the infusion, fill a quart jar one-third full with dried oat-straw herb (available at health-food stores). Pour in boiling water, tighten lid, and allow the solution to steep for at least four hours. Strain and refrigerate the liquid. You can drink it warm or cold. Then you can really start horsing around.

4. **Oysters:** This classic aphrodisiac may actually deserve its reputation. Shellfish (in fact, all seafood) is packed with minerals that are critical components of sex hormones. Minerals are also vital for optimal functioning of your brain and nervous system.

The minerals in seafood are already in their so-called salt forms, which makes them readily usable by the body.

5. **Kelp:** Seaweed is another source of minerals. It is high in iodine, which helps with thyroid function, and it is not uncommon for people suffering a loss of libido to have a mild case of hypothyroidism that doesn't show up in medical tests. If this is the case, kelp can help — though it might take a month or more of regular kelp-eating to feel results. Try eating more Japanese food or sprinkling dried kelp over salads or rice. That might even help make your partner yelp in bed.

6. **Chocolate:** Isn't it great when a food you love is also good for your love life? Chocolates contain methylxanthines, which stimulate the transmission and conduction of nerve impulses. In addition, they also create a feeling of satisfaction. Chocolate is also known as an organoleptic food, which means that its sensual texture, colour, and scent help get you in the mood. Other sensual foods include cocoa, chocolate sauce, ice cream, cheese sauces, and cream sauces. No dope, however, is available about our Indian *mithais*. But judging by India's population figures, they seem to be working pretty well too.

7. **Eggs:** Chockful of B vitamins, especially B6 and B5 (pantothenic acid), eggs can help blow away bedroom blues by balancing hormone levels, maintaining energy levels, and helping the body cope with stress.

Well, try these out and tell me if they work. If they do, who knows, I might even start an Orgasm Café section in my office.

39

Masturbation Facts

I am often asked why I never write about or mention masturbation in my columns, considering that it is so widespread and that I must be seeing so many masturbation-related problems among my patients. To this, I reply that I have colleagues who specialise in writing about masturbation and have been writing about little else for several decades and that I would like to leave this to them.

One day, however, a friend told me, 'Yeah boss, but the same stuff keeps appearing *ad nauseam ad infinitum*. We are told that masturbation does not cause weakness, not to worry, and that the vagina and the clenched fist are very analogous, and that semen is not manufactured from blood. This is only myth exploding. Even I can write such stuff. But what about other scientific facts about masturbation?'

He had a point. So, here are a few Frequently Asked Questions & Answers about masturbation.

What is masturbation?

Masturbation is the self-stimulation of the genitals to achieve sexual arousal and pleasure, usually to the point of orgasm (sexual climax). It is commonly done by touching, stroking or massaging the penis or clitoris until an orgasm is achieved. Some women also use stimulation of the vagina or 'sex toys', such as a vibrator. Men can use some amazing things too. I remember when I was a surgical resident I had to take a guy into the operation theatre and put him under anaesthesia because his penis was stuck in the hole of a hammer's head! It took us a long time and some really skilled manoeuvring to get the thing out in one piece.

Who masturbates?

Just about everybody. Masturbation is a very common practice, even among people who have regular sexual relations with a partner. In one US study, ninety-five per cent of males and eighty-nine per cent of females reported that they have masturbated. Masturbation is the first sexual act experienced by most males and females. In young children, masturbation is a normal part of the growing child's exploration of his or her body. In fact, studies of the unborn human foetus have shown that even unborn children masturbate. Most people continue to masturbate in adulthood, and many do so throughout their lives. So cheer up, you're not the only one.

Why do people masturbate?

In addition to feeling good, masturbation is a good way of relieving the sexual tension that can build up over time, especially for people without partners or whose partners are not willing or available for sex. Masturbation also is a safe sexual alternative for people who wish to avoid pregnancy and the dangers of sexually transmitted diseases. It is also necessary when a man must give a semen sample for infertility testing or for sperm donation. When sexual dysfunction is present in an adult, masturbation may be prescribed by a sex therapist to allow a person to experience an orgasm (often in women) or to delay its arrival (often in men).

Is masturbation normal?

While it once was regarded as a perversion and a sign of a mental disease, masturbation now is regarded as a normal, healthy sexual activity that is pleasant, fulfilling, acceptable, and safe. It is a good way to experience sexual pleasure and can be practised throughout life. Masturbation is only considered a problem when it inhibits sexual activity with a partner, is done in public, or causes significant distress to the person, like when it is done compulsively and/or interferes with daily life and activities.

Is masturbation harmful?

In general, the modern medical community considers masturbation to be a natural and harmless expression of sexuality for both men and women (though there are still some archaic doctors out there). It does not cause any physical injury or harm to the body, and can be performed in moderation throughout a person's lifetime as a part of normal sexual behaviour. Some cultures and religions oppose the use of masturbation or even label it as sinful. This can lead to guilt or shame about the behaviour.

Some experts suggest that masturbation can actually improve sexual health and relationships. By exploring your own body through masturbation, you can determine what is erotically pleasing to you and can share this with your partner. Some partners use mutual masturbation to discover techniques for a more satisfying sexual relationship and to add to their mutual intimacy.

I know what you're thinking. No one seems to be watching, so what are you waiting for?

Go for it!

Appendix

Table I

Types of Impotence

Primary	Impotent since birth
Secondary	Impotence sets in after years of normal sex
Functional	Psychological (10 - 20 %)
Organic	Physical (80 - 90 %)

Causes of Secondary Impotence

1. Diabetes mellitus
2. Hypertension (high blood pressure)
3. Atherosclerosis
4. Renal (kidney) failure
5. Cardiovascular disease
6. Neurological disorders: multiple sclerosis, stroke, paraplegia, spinal cord lesions, Parkinsonism, etc.
7. Sudden injuries, e.g. spinal, pelvic and perineal
8. Gradual injuries, as in bicycle-riders etc.
9. Surgery — operations on bowel, rectum, bladder, retroperitoneum, spine, urethra, prostate etc.

10. Local, e.g. Peyronie's disease, penile curvature, epispadias, hypospadias
11. Medication, e.g. drugs administered for duodenal ulcer, hypertension, mental disease etc.

Table II
Diagnosis of Impotence (ED)

Detailed history-taking and examination
Penile Doppler/ultrasound
The Rigiscan test
Dynamic Infusion Cavernosometry and Cavernosography
Phalloarteriography
Endocrinological evaluation (including hormonal assays)
Neurological evaluation (biothesiometry, corpus cavernosum electromyography)
Psychological assessment
Other special tests

Table III
Treatment Options for Impotence (ED)

Oral Drugs: Viagra, Levitra, Cialis, others
Injection therapy: prostaglandin, phentolamine, papaverine, others Vacuum therapy
Surgery: penile prosthetic implantation, microvascular arterial and venous surgery, surgery for Peyronie's disease, penile curvatures, deformities etc.
Psychotherapy and counseling.